A Pocket Guide to Risk Assessment and Management in Mental Health

Risk assessment and risk management are top of every mental health trust's agenda. This concise and easy-to-read book provides an informative and practical guide to the process of undertaking a risk assessment, arriving at a formulation and then developing a risk management plan.

Covering everything a practitioner may have to think about when undertaking risk assessments in an accessible, logical form, the book includes practice recommendations rooted in the latest theory and evidence base. Attractively presented, plentiful clinical tip boxes, tables, diagrams and case examples make it easy to identify key information. Samples of authentic dialogue demonstrate ways in which to formulate questions and think about complex problems with the person being assessed. A series of accompanying professionally made films, based on actual case studies, are available on a companion website and further illustrate key risk assessment and management skills.

This accessible guidebook is designed for all mental health professionals, and professionals-in-training. It will also be a useful reference for healthcare practitioners who regularly come into contact with people experiencing mental health problems.

Chris Hart is a Senior Lecturer at Kingston University and St George's, University of London, UK and retired nurse consultant for South West London and St George's Mental Health NHS Trust. He has extensive experience in the areas of forensic psychiatry, liaison psychiatry and psychiatric intensive care and has taught risk assessment to a wide range of health professionals, from consultant psychiatrists to paramedics, over the past decade.

A Pocket Guide to Risk Assessment and Management in Mental Health

Chris Hart

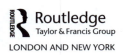

Routledge
Taylor & Francis Group

LONDON AND NEW YORK

First published 2014
by Routledge
2 Park Square, Milton Park, Abingdon, Oxon OX14 4RN

and by Routledge
711 Third Avenue, New York, NY 10017

Routledge is an imprint of the Taylor & Francis Group, an informa business

© 2014 Chris Hart

British Library Cataloguing in Publication Data
A catalogue record for this book is available from the British Library

Library of Congress Cataloging-in-Publication Data
Hart, Christopher, 1956- author.
A pocket guide to risk assessment and management in mental health / Chris Hart.
p. ; cm.
Includes bibliographical references.
I. Title.
[DNLM: 1. Mental Disorders--diagnosis--Handbooks. 2. Mental Disorders--therapy--Handbooks. 3. Mental Health--Handbooks. 4. Risk Assessment--Handbooks. 5. Risk Management--Handbooks. WM 34]
RC454.4
616.89--dc23
2013020818

ISBN13: 978-0-415-70258-4 (hbk)
ISBN13: 978-0-415-70259-1 (pbk)
ISBN13: 978-0-203-79559-0 (ebk)

Typeset in Frutiger
by Saxon Graphics Ltd, Derby

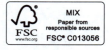

Printed and bound in Great Britain by
TJ International Ltd, Padstow, Cornwall

Contents

List of illustrations   vii
The accompanying films for the Pocket Guide   ix
Acknowledgements   xi

Introduction
About this guide   1
Cultural diversity   6
Gender and sexuality   6
A note about terminology   6

Part 1 Risk assessment – an overview   **9**
Introduction   9
Key issues to determine from a risk assessment   10
Organisational issues and risk assessment and
    risk management   14
Risk of suicide and self-harm   17
Risk of dangerousness, violence and/or homicide   31
Developing a common language for assessing and
    communicating risk   37

Part 2 General principles of risk assessment   **47**
Different approaches to risk assessment   48
Making use of the information gained from assessment   49
Translating the assessment into a formulation   51
The safety of the clinician and patient   51
Taking a referral   54

Part 3 Undertaking a risk assessment   **59**
First impressions   59
Initial communications and developing a rapport   61
Key interview skills   68
Other interview techniques   74
Things to avoid   89
Closing, or finishing, the assessment interview   91
Risk assessment in the context of a full mental health
    assessment   93

Defining the risk   110
Short assessments and re-assessments – the key principles   127
Developing a formulation   129

Part 4   Managing risk   **135**
Introduction   135
Mental capacity   136
Negotiating and writing a care plan for the purposes of
   risk management   139
Therapeutic risk-taking or positive risk management   155
Relapse profiles and crisis plans   158
Record keeping and good documentation   161

Summary and conclusions   **165**

Index   167

Illustrations

Figures

1.1	Psychological states and potential self-harm	19
1.2	Male suicides 2006–2010 per 100,000 of the population by age	25
1.3	Female suicides 2006–2010 per 100,000 of the population by age	25
1.4	Factors affecting current suicide risk	29
2.1	The formula for risk management	50
3.1	The relationship between the degree of collaboration and the risk management plan	63
3.2	Johari's Window adapted for risk	111

Tables

1.1	Key issues to identify during a risk assessment	13
1.2	Suicide rates (per 100,000) by gender, United Kingdom and Northern Ireland, 1955–2009	25
1.3	Number of suicides (per 100,000) by age group and gender for the United Kingdom and Northern Ireland, 2009	25
1.4	The most common methods people use for killing themselves	27
1.5	Clinical risk indicators for suicide	28
1.6	Groups with the highest risk of suicide	30
1.7	United Kingdom homicide rates, 1959–2011	34
1.8	Risk factors in aggression and/or violence	36
1.9	An example of definitions of risk levels	39
2.1	Safety and the referral process	51
3.1	Information to provide to the patient at the start of the assessment	61
3.2	Putting the person at ease with your non-verbal communication and physical presence	68
3.3	Closing the session – key points	92
3.4	Risk and the Mental State Examination [MSE]	103
3.5	Questions to address potential risk and assist in scenario planning	115
3.6	Formulating the risk	130
4.1	A framework for a risk management plan	140
4.2	Structuring a care plan	147

Boxes

1	Case study – William	3
2	Case study – Michael	4
3	The principles of risk assessment	10
4	Frequent findings from inquiries into suicide and homicide	16
5	Key interview skills	69
6	Occurrences that should prompt a re-assessment of risk	129
7	A checklist for teams and patients when working with positive risk management	157
8	A sample relapse profile	158
9	Ten tips for good record keeping	162

The accompanying films for the *Pocket Guide*

Several years ago the Head of Clinical Risk for the South West London and St George's Mental Health NHS Trust, Justin O'Brien, asked me to contribute to a unique project. It was to produce a series of films that would explore a range of risk assessment techniques in different scenarios, featuring interactions between mental health patients and clinicians.

The scripts would be written by staff working in the relevant clinical areas, who would then work with professional actors, directors and production crew to create films that could be used for education and training in this extremely complex area.

In fact, most of the scripts were written by Justin and myself, sometimes with the help of colleagues, but all were based on actual incidents or interactions with patients. Some of the films include a part that demonstrates 'poor practice', often based on what had happened that had brought the incident to people's attention. Crucial to the making of the films was that they were credible and that the skills demonstrated in the 'good practice' section were achievable by the viewing audience.

Making the films was both fascinating and great fun. The director for all of them, Andrew Calloway, was very gifted and always managed to capture the key clinical concerns, as if he had been working in mental health all his career. The actors, provided by Cath Hamilton, were always of the highest calibre, bringing such an air of authenticity that people watching would often ask if they were actually nurses or doctors, or even patients.

The two films featured on the website to complement the text in the *Pocket Guide* came out of that work but are very different in their subject matter. One focuses on the risk of suicide while the other explores a serious assault carried out on a clinician by a person who is very psychotic. The first film has a section that shows poor practice, followed by a longer interview demonstrating how a relatively inexperienced nurse can carefully assess the person's risk in the context of his changed mental state. The second film explores danger to others, often thought to be 'unpredictable' by many clinicians working with people experiencing mental health problems. This film is staged very differently, showing a violent assault on a member of staff by a patient, then giving the viewer the opportunity to look for triggers and indications that it was likely to occur. The final part of the film features a lengthy interview with the patient, after the assault has occurred, during which his rationale for the assault emerges.

Much of the material from parts 3 and 4 of the *Pocket Guide* links directly to the films. Although there is sample dialogue in the book, the films on the website demonstrate the techniques highlighted in the text in a wholly different way, with the viewer able to look for the non-verbal cues and the human dynamic between interviewer and interviewee. When Justin and I have used these films in teaching practice, course participants have always cited them as crucial learning. I hope that, in accessing them on the website and using the materials and exercises that go with them, you will find the films equally rewarding.

 To access the companion website please visit http://www. routledge.com/cw/hart, and use the scratch-off access code located on the inside front cover.

Acknowledgements

The work in this book is completely influenced by the many gifted and learned clinicians I've worked with over the years. I'm particularly grateful to my old colleagues in the Assessment & Treatment Team in Lambeth, the Liaison Psychiatry Service at St George's Hospital, including David, Dru, Paul, Rachel, Marcus and Jyoti. I was extremely fortunate to work with some wonderful clinicians in the Intensive Care and Forensic teams at Springfield Hospital, especially Gavin, Teresa, Mary, Sallie, Davis, Alex, Jimmy and Palmer. I've also benefited from working alongside the very talented mental health team at Kingston University. I had help from my nurse consultant colleagues, especially Barrie Green, Alan Howard and Ian Higgins. However, I would be negligent if I did not pay very special tribute to Justin O'Brien and Tony McGranaghan, both expert nurses in their own fields, great teachers and collaborators to whom I'm eternally grateful. Many of their ideas, advice and experiences are woven into the fabric of this work. The book is dedicated to the many patients with whom I have had the privilege of working over a long career.

Introduction

About this Guide

The principle aim of this *Pocket Guide* is to provide a brief, practical guide to the process of undertaking a risk assessment, arriving at a formulation and, from that, developing a risk management plan.

It is designed to be used as an *aide memoire* and a prompt for clinicians in the workplace undertaking mental health risk assessments, including those working in non mental health settings. However, it is also applicable as a foundation to risk assessment in specialist settings, such as forensic services. Although set out in clearly defined sections, it is important to remember that the practice of sitting down with someone and having this discussion will not necessarily reproduce the linear structure here. Indeed, one of the most important skills in undertaking risk assessments is the ability to 'go with' the person and her/his story, while retaining an internal structure that enables you to address all the pertinent issues and fully assess risk during the course of the interview.

This is not an academic text that will provide in-depth information about suicide, self-harm or other risk behaviours. Nor is it aimed at providing a theoretical discourse about risk assessment. Its practice recommendations are rooted in the latest theory and evidence base and there is also a reading list to provide additional information and more background theory. The main purpose of the *Pocket Guide* is for it to be used in clinical situations and be of practical help. In this context, the statistics and other information contained in Part 1 are not there to be viewed in isolation but integrated into the assessment process, helping you think about your patient in the wider context, and applying known clinical risk indicators and statistical information to the individual whom you are assessing. For example, it is known a man aged between 35 and 54, recently separated from his partner, unemployed and depressed is statistically at risk of experiencing suicidal thoughts and acting upon them. This doesn't tell you that the 52-year-old man you are assessing will try and kill himself, but indicates there are specific risk factors to be taken into account that should inform your assessment.

While the *Pocket Guide* acknowledges the importance of other forms of risk, e.g. self neglect, it will focus mainly on risk to self, in the form of self-harm and suicide, and to others in the form of violence and aggression.

Although it largely describes a collaborative process at all stages, it also recognises that more restrictive and coercive approaches are sometimes necessary, e.g. where concern about safety is not shared between the assessor and person being assessed and the assessor's concerns to manage risk outweigh the requirements of a collaborative approach.

The *Pocket Guide* does not recommend or directly address the use of 'risk assessment tools', screening tools or other recognised tools for assessing such things as psychosis, depression and anxiety etc. There are several reasons for this: there will be guidance about how to use these with the tools themselves; different health organisations advocate the use of different tools and the tools themselves are, inevitably, of varying quality. Validated risk assessment or screening tools can be useful – and you may also use other assessment tools to assist in the risk assessment process, exploring depression, anxiety or psychosis for instance – and their use is recommended where applicable. A significant advantage to using recognised assessment tools, particularly those related to risk, is that they provide a common language, specific prompts and structure, and they force the clinician to ask questions, some of which might be quite difficult. However, any tool is only as effective in assessing risk as the clinician using it and completing it should not distract from the overall process of assessment described here. In particular, the person being interviewed should not feel s/he is being subjected to a 'tick box process'.

In the latter part of the book, two particular case studies are used to illustrate different skills and particular areas of risk assessment (see Boxes 1 and 2 below). The extracts cited here are based on actual people who were assessed and treated, but anonymised and adapted to maintain confidentiality. One case study focuses on a 35-year-old man who is experiencing suicidal thoughts in the community. Later, he is in discussion with a clinician after a suicide attempt, having ingested paracetamol tablets.[1] The second features a young man who is in hospital following a serious assault in the context of a psychotic disorder. In both cases, the details of the individual's background rarely feature as prominent issues in the risk assessment as the conversation focuses on more immediate matters relating to the risks facing each person. However, it always provides a context for the current situation and informs the clinician's responses.

You will note the reference to terms such as discussion and conversation in the above paragraph, while the overall task being described is that of a risk assessment. One of the skills the *Pocket Guide* will try to convey is the way in which an assessment can be conducted in a conversational way. While this may take slightly longer, it is likely to help the clinician develop a better relationship and elicit more information. Nonetheless, while there may be quite a distinct style, or 'voice', in the clinical examples within the *Pocket Guide* it is necessary to remember that every clinician needs to find her or his own voice and style rather than trying to remember a certain question or way of seeking information seen elsewhere.

The *Pocket Guide* is broken into four parts. Part 1 contains an overview of the risk assessment process and information related to risk assessment and risk management, including clinical risk indicators; Part 2 looks at different approaches to risk assessment and its general principles; Part 3 focuses on the process of, and skills needed for, undertaking a risk assessment; Part 4 concentrates on risk management.

Finally, it is crucial to remind ourselves that, no matter how comprehensive and competent the assessment, risk can never be wholly eliminated. Rather, clinicians are engaged in risk minimisation in a dynamic process, with the level of engagement from the person involved in the assessment crucial to its outcome.

Box 1: Case study – William

(See clinical examples, in Part 3: Undertaking a risk assessment)

William is a 35-year-old man. He has recently separated from his partner, Kelly. This followed a difficult relationship in which he had become increasingly dependent on her, having been made redundant from his job in information technology. Since she left, he has struggled financially, with a recent cut in his benefits, and he is facing the prospect of losing his flat and having to move back to live with his mother.

His father died a year ago after a long illness and William has found it difficult to come to terms with his loss. William's father, a quantity surveyor, was always an important figure in his life, although William did not think they had a particularly close relationship, certainly not as close a relationship as William's brother had with their father. He has few close friends though lots of acquaintances from work and college, and has never been able to confide in others. He and his brother are close but William feels he always has to live up to his brother's achievements and never wants to appear 'weak' or unable to cope in his eyes. William has always experienced his mother as rather aloof and distant, though he says they have a good relationship.

William has only taken cannabis on a few occasions, in his late teens. He has no history of alcohol abuse but, as he began to feel unable to cope with the mounting stress he was experiencing, began drinking more. He says when he is stressed, he cannot think clearly and feels the need to 'escape', finding both his feelings and the sense of 'crowded thoughts' too difficult to bear. He has stopped doing things like yoga, reading and socialising, which he was doing until a few weeks before Kelly left.

Over the past five to six weeks he has had trouble getting off to sleep, and then waking through the night. His appetite is diminished, he has trouble concentrating and is not enjoying the sorts of things he used to. He can see no hope for the future and is convinced no one would miss him if he were no longer there. Unable to think clearly about things like paying his bills or looking after his flat, he can see no way out of his situation.

In the clinical examples we initially meet William at home and then there are examples of discussion with him after he has been admitted to an acute psychiatric ward following an attempt to kill himself.

Box 2: Case study – Michael

(See clinical examples, in Part 3: Undertaking a risk assessment)

Michael is currently an inpatient on an acute psychiatric ward, having been admitted after assaulting someone in an apparently unprovoked attack in the street. He was initially arrested by the police but was so psychotic he was then brought to hospital under Section 136 of the Mental Health Act. This was converted to a Section 2 after he was assessed. Now in his late thirties, he has a history of psychotic illness, with several lengthy admissions to hospital.

Michael experienced his first episode of psychosis three months after starting university. He had grown up in a small town in Sussex but moved with his mother to London when he was 11 after she left Michael's father. His father had been a successful commercial artist but suffered from a psychotic illness and was a heavy drinker, prone to violence when he had been drinking. He died just before Michael's eighteenth birthday. Michael's mother had several partners in the period after separating from her husband and Michael claims one of them was violent and possibly sexually abusive, though this has never been substantiated. He now says that the same man has visited him in hospital and 'done things'.

Over the past five years, Michael has become increasingly isolated. Once keen on cricket and football, he has lost interest in most things. He doesn't see his old friends and rarely associates with anyone other than people he has met in hospital. He regularly smokes cannabis and has used a variety of other illicit drugs including cocaine, ecstasy and amphetamines. His illicit drug use is usually associated with a relapse in his mental state.

Michael understands his experiences as being the result of him having special powers and being different to other people. However, he also feels vulnerable to what he terms 'being infected' by other people. His definition of this phenomenon varies but he often describes it as people being able to put thoughts in his head, change the way he feels and control him in unpleasant ways. It has been observed that this phenomenon usually seems to occur when he is feeling physically and psychologically aroused, anxious and/or angry. He will often ruminate on things that have been said and, when he is doing this, isolate himself and not communicate with others.

Michael has been described as experiencing paranoid delusions, auditory hallucinations, ideas of reference and thought insertion. He presents as a risk to others on the ward, having made threats of physical violence to fellow patients and nurses, as well as punching and kicking another patient.

Cultural diversity

It isn't possible to detail all the variations in cultural diversity that could impact on a risk assessment. These have to be an essential part of your assessment. If you are assessing someone about whose culture you have little understanding, it is important to endeavour to find out any information that will help you arrive at a clear formulation and to make clear, safe clinical decisions. Equally, if language is a barrier, you should seek the assistance of a professional interpreter (it is inadvisable to use a carer/friend or to find someone 'who speaks the language' to undertake such a complex task unless conducting an emergency assessment with no opportunity to arrange the assistance of an interpreter).

Gender and sexuality

Again, it isn't impossible to explore in great detail the variety of gender issues relevant to the risk assessment process within the space of the *Pocket Guide*, nor those related to sexual orientation. In Part 1 there are detailed statistics that delineate risks for different groups and there will be occasional references to specific risk factors, e.g. sexual abuse and its relationship to self-harm. However, most sections of the *Pocket Guide* will help you think about accessing specific risks and exploring different risk indicators through the assessment process with a view to making that assessment completely relevant to the individual, regardless of gender or sexual orientation.

A note about terminology

Different terms are used in any number of different settings for and about the people who use or come into contact with mental health services. The most important element to communicate about the assessment process is that it is an exchange between two people and it will always be easier if the clinician remembers that.

While there are different rationales for preferring each term, I shall talk about people, the person and the individual in most cases, but use the term patient when necessary as there is evidence that people using mental health services prefer to be described as patients rather than clients, service users or customers (Barker 2003; Simmons *et al.* 2010; McGuire-Sneickus *et al.* 2003).

References

Barker, P. (2003) 'Assessment in Practice', in Barker, P. (ed.) *Psychiatric and Mental Health Nursing: The Craft of Caring.* London: Hodder Arnold.

McGuire-Sneickus, R., McCabe, R. and Preibe, S. (2003) 'Patient, client or service user? A survey of patient preferences in dress and address of six mental health professions', *Psychiatric Bulletin*, 27: 305–08.

Simmons, P., Hawley, C.J., Gale, T.M. and Sivakumaram, T. (2010) 'Service user, patient, client, user or survivor: describing recipients of mental health services', *The Psychiatrist*, 34: 20–23.

Note

1   In each clinical example, reference is made only to a 'clinician'. This is because the skills and risk assessments illustrated here could be conducted by a variety of mental health and non mental health clinicians, rather than just psychiatrists or mental health nurses.

Part 1: Risk assessment – an overview

Assessment, in the context of mental health, refers to the process of gathering and analysing information from multiple and diverse sources, including a semi-structured interview with the person concerned, in order to develop an understanding and evaluation of a possible mental health problem (see Box 3 below).

It is the fundamental starting point for any process of care. It determines the clinician's understanding of the issues the patient wishes to address, as well as the clinician's concerns about the person, which that person may not share. Moreover, it presents an opportunity to listen to the person's story, their account of themselves. This, with the exploration of strengths, coping strategies, problems and/or needs is a key part of establishing a rapport with the person, which is essential when risk needs to be assessed. Considering all elements of risk is an integral part of the overall assessment process.

Risk is a neutral occurrence but with an implied possibility of loss or hazard. In the context of mental health, it has been described as:

> The likelihood of behaviour (or situations) that may be harmful or beneficial to oneself or to others. Risk assessment involves analysing potential outcomes of this behaviour (or situation); and risk management involves devising a care plan to minimize harmful behaviour and maximise beneficial behaviour.
>
> (Callaghan and Waldcock 2006)

The *Pocket Guide* works on the basis that it is far more effective to use discussion in the form of a semi-structured interview as the basis for the clinician's approach rather than a 'checklist approach' (Alderdice *et al.* 2010). It also recognises that some people who either go on to harm themselves or others or are experiencing ideas about risk behaviours, e.g. attempting suicide, will verbally deny them, thus necessitating the very rigorous, inquisitive and holistic methodology detailed here. Above all, it should be remembered that risk is:

- a dynamic process – different elements can change, changing the risks and their impact on the patient;
- context dependent – what is 'risky' in one context may not be in another;
- subject to the influence of the clinician – as soon as the clinician intervenes through the process of an assessment, that will affect the risk. While we would hope that it will begin to minimise it, there is the possibility that, in addressing one risk, another arises (see below).

Most importantly, as has already been emphasised, we must remember that no matter how good the risk assessment, risk cannot be eliminated, only minimised.

Risk behaviours are influenced by:

- the patient's own psychopathology and individual situation;
- a range of clinical risk factors (see the 'Organisational issues and risk assessment and risk management' and 'Risk of suicide and self-harm', page 14 and 28);
- any crisis in external relationships, e.g. with family members or the clinical team;
- the context in which the person is acting.

Box 3: The principles of risk assessment

- Gathering and analysing information.
- Taking a rigorous approach – involving the multi-disciplinary team wherever possible.
- Matching the time to the potential seriousness of the situation or using the available time to gather the essential information.
- Adopting as collaborative an approach as possible.
- Communicating the risk effectively and clearly.
- Using a shared model understood by all members of the clinical team and communicated to potential referrers.

Key issues to determine from a risk assessment

Key information can be acquired from the patient through their own history and from interviews with them and others. Past risk behaviours and past risk history are good indicators of current risk. It is essential to look at past incidents and consider the nature of the incident, specifically and accurately. For example, what harm was caused? What were the background circumstances of the incident? Who suffered harm? What risk factors were present at the time? It is also important to explore what was going on in the patient's life at the time.

As well as identifying all possible risks, i.e. to the person her/himself and/or others, it is essential to have determined at the conclusion of even a brief risk assessment the following (also see Table 1.1):

Recentness
How recently did the event occur? Where recent incidents have occurred the current risk must be seen as greater than if it were an isolated incident. However, it is vital to review the current situation in the context of the entire risk history for the person you're with, even if the last incident was a considerable time ago or the circumstances initially appear to be different.

Immediacy
You should try to establish how immediate the risk is. If there doesn't appear to be any current risks, what would change to make *potential* risks *actual* risks or, if recent risks are no longer current, what has changed to bring this about?

Severity
The more serious the potential consequences of an incident, the more robust you will need to be in addressing it, even if the person is reluctant to engage, tries to assure you there is no longer any risk, or other clinicians have not appeared concerned.

Patterns
When undertaking the assessment you should be looking for common patterns that lead to an incident occurring, including anything in the person's relapse profile or risk history.

Intent

Rather than accepting the actual consequences of the person's actions, which may not have been particularly harmful, it is essential to explore her/his intent.

For example:

• Although an overdose of the actual medication taken could not have been lethal, the person may not have known this and still intended to kill themselves by taking it.
• An individual may have been prevented from harming someone else, or not inflicted significant harm in an assault. However, this cannot be presumed to reveal the person's actual intent. You should still explore thoroughly what s/he would have done had the opportunity been there to complete the assault uninterrupted or, now they have been thwarted, what they would do if they got another opportunity. Moreover, if there is any intention to harm a specific individual, that person should be informed at the earliest opportunity and, if appropriate, the police should also be informed.

Current intent is one of the strongest indicators of future behaviour.

Frequency

The more frequent the incidents, the greater the risk and the more robust the assessor needs to be in addressing it.

Warning signs

How would anyone know things were getting worse?

Plan

The level of planning by the patient prior to carrying out a behaviour is an indicator of both the intent and the broader elements of risk to be managed and should be explored thoroughly, including:

• When did the person first start thinking about doing something dangerous to themselves or others?
• What options did s/he consider for doing this?
• How did s/he rule things out and come to her/his final choice of means of acting?
• When did this become a 'plan' that s/he knew s/he would act on?

- How many things had to be done to put the plan into action, for example, looking on internet sites for information about potential lethality, buying tablets, waiting for the opportunity to be alone?
- Had other things been done, e.g. the person putting her/his affairs in order, getting pets looked after?
- Had the person had to actively deceive others to carry out the plan, e.g. telling them they were going to be doing something else, go somewhere else that would have appeared to be safe?
- How long was the plan in place before being acted upon?
- Was there anything specific that led the person to initiate the plan at the time s/he did?

Level of collaboration

How likely is the person to work with any risk management plan? How is the individual's willingness to collaborate influenced by issues such as capacity, insight/awareness and attitude to treatment?

Table 1.1   Key issues to identify during a risk assessment.

Who?	Who is the person(s) at risk?
What?	What is the specific risk(s) – please name each risk identified.
When?	When is the person at risk, e.g. now? In the future – what would change to increase or minimise the risk? If the person was assessed as previously being at risk but is not now – **what has changed?**
Where?	Where would the person be safe, e.g. does the person need to be in a more restrictive environment or seen more frequently?
Why?	Why is the person currently vulnerable to these risks?
How?	How collaborative is the person likely to be with any risk management plan?
WHAT IS THE PLAN TO ADDRESS EACH CURRENT AND POTENTIAL RISK? Has it been documented? Has it been communicated?	

Key clinical tip

A comprehensive risk assessment carefully considers the 'What if?' questions, e.g. what if something happens that might affect the risk, what would the person do in certain situations? If this highlights potential, as opposed to actual, risk it should lead to **contingency planning** to address those potential situations.

Organisational issues and risk assessment and risk management

The *Pocket Guide* cannot address team functioning and organisation in depth but it is worth considering some key organisational, team and individual issues that increase the effectiveness of risk assessment and management – and, conversely, can cause inordinate problems if ignored or presented as a problem.

Organisational factors that can undermine effective risk assessment and risk management

A crucial starting point is organisations that have inadequate policies both for risk assessment and risk management itself. Equally damaging is the failure to have coherent and robust policies that reflect the real, lived experience of staff engaged in work where they will be undertaking these tasks, e.g. lone working, home visits. Organisations should also not make the mistake of thinking that having a policy in place, however good, means it has fulfilled its responsibilities and that all will be well. There should be a confidence borne out of experience that the policies are effective in influencing practice and are helpful to staff in their clinical practice. Other factors include:

- conflicting service demands, e.g. waiting times for admissions/bed pressures;
- staffing shortages or lack of resources;
- caseloads that do not allow sufficient time for good practice;
- poor clinical environments;

- contemporary models and thinking not accommodating the patient's needs, e.g. specialist services excluding patients/moving people from one service or team to another for organisational rather than clinical reasons.

Team factors that can undermine effective risk assessment and risk management

- Systematic risk assessment not undertaken.
- Risk indicators denied or minimised by responsible professionals.
- Clinical responsibility not clearly defined or transferred appropriately.
- Poor communication internally and with other agencies.
- Poor liaison with other agencies.
- Inadequate support to clinicians managing patients with immediate risk.

Individual factors that can undermine effective risk assessment and risk management

- The experience, capability and attitudes of the clinician.
- Workload, time and external pressures.
- The emotional and psychological capacity to manage difficult work at any one time.

It is important to recognise that all of these factors will vary over time and be affected by a variety of internal and external influences (Harrison and Hart 2006).

Addressing individual and structural deficits
Key principles
1. Building effective, well managed and well led teams that work together is crucial.
2. Ongoing education and training are required.
3. Organisations have to be committed to prioritising the management of identified risks rather than trying to manage risk within a pre-determined budget.
4. Those with the responsibility to manage risk must also have the authority to make decisions.
5. Other disciplines need to understand the nursing experience on inpatient units and respond to it, e.g. listening to dynamic risk changes, views on prescribing, levels of observation etc.

Other factors

1. Provide skills-based training and education programmes that integrate theory with the realities of practice.
2. Provide individual and team clinical supervision that addresses caseloads/patient allocation at least monthly, giving staff safe forums for thinking and talking about patients.
3. Develop work practices that increase emotional intelligence.
4. Resources have to be made available to manage risk – there is a huge incentive for clinicians not to 'reveal' risk if they are expected to manage it without the necessary support and resource.
5. Barriers to rapid assessment have to be removed.
6. Accessible and responsive services have to be more than an aspiration.
7. Services should be designed with cohesive risk management as the main priority.
8. The culture of saying 'no' to referrers has to be eradicated.
9. Develop organisational models that support risk assessment.
10. Have defined clinical models of care for inpatient units.
11. Develop strong relational management – improve staff-management relations and staff input into decision making.
12. Bridge the gap between the managerial/business ideology and clinical culture (Harrison and Hart 2006).

Common findings from inquiries

If any of the factors listed in Box 4 are present in a case with which you are working, they should alert you to potentially serious problems.

Box 4: Frequent findings from inquiries into suicide and homicide

Confusion over diagnosis.
Episodes viewed in isolation.
Delays or inappropriate responses.
Poor record keeping.
Poor inter-agency co-ordination.
Poor communication between agencies.
Not acknowledging family/carer concerns.
Lack of clarity about confidentiality.
Training specific to risk is lacking.
Non-compliance with treatment plans (often not addressed).
Lack of face-to-face contact with the patient.

(Appleby *et al.* 2006)

Risk of suicide and self-harm

Key definitions

There are, in fact, no universally agreed definitions for suicide and what is sometimes termed attempted suicide. The reality of understanding the acts described below is that they are often far more complex than these definitions allow. However, in order to develop a more general understanding, unambiguous and widely understood terms are useful.

Self-harm

This has been described as a non-fatal act, carried out deliberately and with the intention to inflict harm, in the form of an acute episode of behaviour by an individual with variable motivation (Gelder *et al.* 2001). Hawton *et al.* (2007) describe it as intentional acts of self-poisoning or self-injury irrespective of the type of motivation or degree of suicidal intent.

Attempted suicide

This involves self-injurious behaviour with varying degrees of suicidal intent with a non-fatal outcome.

Parasuicide

Although commonly used, this is a term that often confuses attempted suicide, self-harm and 'a cry for help'. Hawton (2005), one of the country's leading experts on the subject, describes it as, '[n]on fatal deliberate self-harm', though most contemporary writers would not now include the term 'deliberate'.

Suicide

This is a self-inflicted act, causing one's own death. Suicide may be direct or indirect. There will be varying degrees of suicidal intent.

Suicide is a *direct act* when an individual takes an action that leads to the loss of her/his own life, e.g. by self-poisoning or hanging, either as an end to be attained, i.e. to be dead, or as a means to another end, as when a person kills her/himself to escape unbearable feelings or a particular situation, or can see no other solution to a set of problems.

Suicide has been described as an *indirect act* when one does not do what is necessary to escape death, such as leaving a burning building, but this would not meet a legal definition.

Self-harm

The phrase 'self-harm' is used to describe a range of things that people do to themselves in an intentional and often hidden way. The act can be premeditated, planned or impulsive. It can involve:

- cutting;
- burning;
- scalding;
- banging or scratching one's own body;
- breaking bones;
- hair pulling;
- swallowing poisonous substances or objects, including prescribed medication and illicit drugs;
- hanging;
- strangulation;
- mutilation of parts of the body;
- interfering with wound healing.

Motives for self-harm will be highly personal or individual and do not necessarily sit within medicalised or biological models. These include:

- a release of tension, frustration or distress;
- to feel and regain control;
- releasing 'bad' feelings;
- to punish oneself;
- to assuage feelings of guilt;
- an incapacity to understand and manage painful feelings;
- as a means of expressing emotional pain.

Thus, the person who is highly aroused may describe themselves as feeling:

- stressed;
- overwhelmed;
- unable to cope;
- hypersensitive.

Conversely, those in a dissociated state may describe themselves as feeling:

- numb;
- empty;
- 'lost';
- disconnected;
- unreal.

Repeated self-harm is often associated with the desire to manage unbearable psychic pain and/or unbearable situations and can include the wish to die (Hjelmeland *et al.* 2002; O'Connor *et al.* 2009a). The physical pain or discomfort that stems from the act can provide distraction and/or a sense of relief.

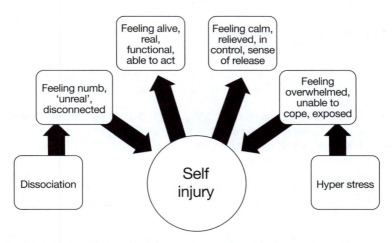

Figure 1.1   Psychological states and potential self-harm, adapted from www.FirstSigns.org

It is important to note that, as with clinical risk indicators (see the 'Clinical risk indicators' section, page 28), the statistics in this section cannot be seen as reliable predictors of individual behaviour. However, they are included here for two reasons.

Firstly, they serve as a reminder of the vulnerability of particular client groups with whom we often feel so familiar that it is easy to underestimate or overlook the risk levels. Secondly, it is important to recognise that there are different risk factors for people with different mental health problems.

For example, self-harm among older people has a distinct and different profile, with suicidal intent often far more prominent. In young people, different forms of self-harm may indicate different intent. Only 40 per cent of those who cut themselves wanted to die, while 66 per cent who self-poisoned had sought death (Alderdice 2010). Reasons among South Asian women will often be very different from white European women (Bhugra and Desai 2002).

Estimates of the numbers of people who self-harm in the UK vary.

- It was the cause for at least 200,000 general hospital presentations in 2010, a rise from 150,000 in 2002 (NHS Information Centre 2012; DoH 2002).
- In the year August 2009 to July 2010:
    - 96,030 people were admitted after intentionally self-poisoning (61 per cent women, 39 per cent men);
    - 7,940 people were admitted having self-harmed with a sharp or blunt object, i.e. cutting (52.5 per cent women and 47.5 per cent men).
- It is estimated that as many as 400 per 100,000 of the population self-harm each year (Horrocks 2002).
- As many as one in ten people may self-harm at some time in their life.
- Repetition of self-harm increases the risk of suicide and at least 15–25 per cent repeat an act of self-harm within a year of their previous incident. Risk of repetition is greatest within the first few weeks of the earlier act and repetition increases the risk of eventual suicide (Hawton 2005; Zahl and Hawton 2004).

These latter statistics should alert all clinicians to the huge risks associated with people who re-present with self-harm about whom it is often felt there is no serious suicide risk, that the person 'isn't serious' or that every presentation is the same and therefore doesn't merit a proper assessment. It needs to be remembered that every time someone presents with self-harm the situation may have changed and there may be a significant risk of them going on to attempt suicide or, indeed, this may have been an occasion when the act was one of suicidal intent rather than self-harm.

Groups experiencing a greater risk of self-harm

These include:

- people who have experienced physical, emotional or sexual abuse during childhood;
- gay and bisexual people, who seem to be more likely to self-harm, as well as other minority groups discriminated against by society (RCP 2006);
- people with pervasive developmental disabilities such as autism will often self-harm;
- people who are depressed or have other significant mental health problems – those with mental health problems are 20 times more likely to self-harm than people in the general population;
- people dependent on drugs or alcohol;
- those facing major life problems or living in very stressful circumstances during times when they feel particularly vulnerable.

Self-harm and young people

- It has been estimated that 7 to 14 per cent of adolescents will self-harm at some time in their life.
- Young women are most likely to self-harm.
- The percentage of young men self-harming is increasing.
- A common factor is a feeling of helplessness or powerlessness with regard to their emotions.

Sexual abuse and self-harm

- The impact of the experience of childhood abuse on adult self-harm is now well established, as are its link with suicidal behaviour, particularly among women (Bebbington *et al.* 2009).
- Where abuse is repeated and sexual abuse was by a member of the immediate family, there is a stronger association with suicide attempts (Brezo *et al.* 2008).
- There is a likelihood of increased risk of self-harm in people with a history of childhood sexual abuse, particularly if the abuse is perpetrated over a long period, the victim knows the perpetrator and forced penetration was used (Cutliffe 2005).

The issue of sexual abuse is important, as can be seen, and could potentially be spoken about by someone during a risk assessment, particularly if the presenting problem is one of self-harm or suicide. Whether or not it is best to explore this in a risk assessment needs careful consideration (see Clinical example 10, page 82).

Prognosis

The commonly expressed view that people who self-harm are either 'not serious' or will not go on to kill themselves is *not* borne out by the evidence. The prognosis following an episode of self-harm is poor:

- The rate of completed suicide in people who have self-harmed in the previous year is 100 times that of the general population.
- 1 per cent will kill themselves in the first year.
- 7 per cent will kill themselves within ten years (NHS Centre for Reviews and Dissemination, 1998).

However, the risk of self-harm escalating, either to further self-harm attempts or suicide attempts, can be offset by offering a psychosocial assessment, as recommended in the NICE Guidelines (NICE 2004). A study of people presenting with self-harm to emergency departments found that a psychosocial assessment reduced the risk of a single repeat episode by 51 per cent in individuals without a history of psychiatric treatment and by 26 per cent in individuals with a history of psychiatric treatment. For those people with a repetition of up to five episodes, a psychosocial assessment decreased the risk of a further episode by 13 per cent (Bergen *et al.* 2010).

Suicide

The relationship between self-harm and suicide is complex. However, although acts of self-harm and suicide attempts do not necessarily involve an intention to die, there is a strong association between self-harm, attempted suicide and subsequent death by suicide. In addition to the statistics above, a British study found that women who have a history of self-harm are 15 times more likely to die by suicide compared with those who do not. The risk is particularly high during the six months following an episode of self-harm.

The precipitating life events for women who attempt suicide tend to be losses or crises in significant social or family relationships. As with men, suicide is more common among women who are single or recently separated, divorced or widowed.

However, women are more likely than men to have stronger social supports, to feel that their relationships are deterrents to suicide, and to seek psychiatric and other medical intervention (Cooper *et al.* 2005; American Foundation for Suicide Prevention 1997).

In terms of trends, suicide rates in women peaked in 1960 and, apart from a reverse in 1980, have been in steady decline since. The trend in suicide rates for men over the past 50 years is different. Twenty years of decline were followed by a sustained increase between 1970 and 1990, by which time it had almost returned to its 1950 level. The 1990s and early twenty-first century saw the numbers falling again before a small increase. While the highest suicide rates fall between the ages of 35 and 54 in both men and women, the increase is much sharper among women than men (see Tables 1.2 and 1.3).

Suicide statistics for England and Wales include the following numbers:

• There are 4,000 to 5,500 suicides per year in England and Wales.
• Approximately 25 per cent of these people have been in recent contact with mental health services.
• Between 160 and 200 psychiatric inpatients die by suicide annually, most commonly by hanging; this figure has fallen during the past decade.
• The suicide rate equates to approximately 1 per cent of UK deaths.
• 75 per cent of all suicide deaths are male. While male deaths from suicide are greater in all age groups, the ratio varies in different age ranges.
• The period of highest risk after discharge from inpatient care is the first 14 days.
• Over one-fifth of individuals dying by suicide have not been adherent to medication in the preceding month and nearly one-third have disengaged from services.

Suicide and young people
• Suicide accounts for almost 23 per cent of all deaths of people aged 15–24 years, and is the second most common cause of death in young people after accidental death (Office for National Statistics 2007).
• As many as 20–45 per cent of older adolescents say they have had suicidal thoughts (Hawton and James 2005).

Table 1.2   Suicide rates (per 100,000) by gender, United Kingdom and Northern Ireland, 1955–2009.

	1950	1955	1960	1965	1970	1975	1980	1985	1990	1995	2000	2005	2009
Total	9.5	10.7	10.7	10.4	7.0	7.5	8.8	9.0	8.1	7.4	7.5	6.7	6.9
Male	12.7	13.6	13.3	12.2	8.4	9.0	11.0	12.4	12.6	11.7	11.8	10.4	10.9
Female	6.5	8.0	8.2	8.7	6.5	6.0	6.7	5.8	3.8	3.2	3.3	3.2	3.0

Table 1.3   Number of suicides (per 100,000) by age group and gender for the United Kingdom and Northern Ireland, 2009.

Age (years)	5–14	15–24	25–34	35–44	45–54	55–64	65–74	74+
All males	0.1	5.1	8.7	11.4	10.8	8.3	5.7	6.0
All females	0.1	7.9	13.9	18.6	17.3	12.7	8.7	10.2
Total	0.1	2.1	3.4	4.3	4.5	4.0	2.9	3.3

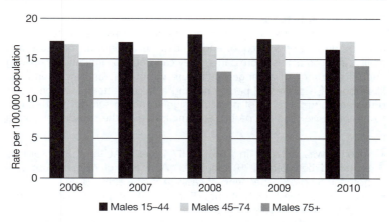

Figure 1.2   Male suicides 2006–10 per 100,000 of the population by age

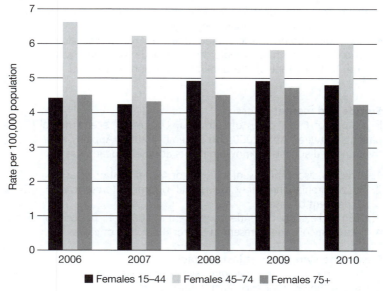

Figure 1.3   Female suicides 2006–10 per 100,000 of the population by age

Suicide and substance misuse

Substance misuse has long been recognised as a risk factor for suicide and suicide attempts. Alcohol and drugs affect thinking and reasoning ability, and can act as depressants. They can decrease inhibitions, making impulsive actions of a dangerous nature more likely and increasing the likelihood of a depressed person making a suicide attempt. Alcohol and drugs are thought to be of particular significance in suicides that appear to be impulsive, and are particularly implicated in the suicides of young men.

• Alcohol was a factor in 785, or 57.1 per cent, of 1,373 suicides examined between 1999 and 2003. A history of drug misuse was noted in 522, or 38 per cent, of cases (Appleby *et al.* 2006).
• Estimates suggest that about 15 per cent of people who misuse alcohol may eventually kill themselves.
• Among people who misuse drugs, the risk of suicide is 20 times that of the general population (Faulkner 1997).
• Men are nine times more likely than women to misuse alcohol. Men diagnosed with alcohol addiction are six times as likely to die by suicide as men in the general population.
• Although women are less likely than men to misuse alcohol, those who do are at a much greater risk of suicide than men, with a suicide rate 20 times that of the general population (Harris and Barraclough 1997).

Suicide and mental illness

In a study of 6,367 cases of suicide by current or recent mental health patients between April 2000 and December 2004 (Appleby *et al.* 2006), the primary diagnosis of known patients at time of death was:

1. Affective disorder (present in 2,821 or 46 per cent of cases).
2. Schizophrenia and other delusional disorders (present in 1,145 or 19 per cent of cases).
3. Drug and alcohol dependence (present in 206 or 11 per cent of cases).
4. Personality disorder (present in 518 or 8 per cent of cases).

Presenting symptoms at last contact

In the same study, the following symptoms were noted to have been present at the last clinical contact before death:

1. Emotional distress (present in 1,971 cases).
2. Depressive illness (present in 1,706 cases).

3. Hopelessness (present in 841 cases).
4. Suicidal ideas (present in 780 cases).
5. Recent self-harm (present in 770 cases).
6. Increased use of alcohol (present in 697 cases).
7. Deterioration in physical health (present in 463 cases).
8. Delusions or hallucinations (present in 427 cases).

Table 1.4   The most common methods people use for killing themselves (DoH 2003)

Males	**%**	**Females**	**%**
Hanging	42	Self-poisoning	48
Self-poisoning	26	Hanging	27
Other	22	Other	15
Jumping	5	Jumping	7
Motor gas	5	Motor gas	5

Clinical risk indicators for suicide

Clinical risk indicators for suicide are factors identified in people who have either killed themselves or attempted suicide. They are derived from large-scale population studies, with researchers looking into cases where individuals have either attempted or completed suicide, and can be used by the assessor as identifying key issues that *may* highlight areas of risk in the individual's background. However, this does not necessarily indicate that someone of male gender, recently unemployed and depressed is going to kill himself. Nor does it indicate that someone who does not have many of these factors in his presentation apart from current suicidal thoughts and intent should not be considered likely to kill himself. Identification of the risk factors highlighted here should occur during a comprehensive assessment and be judged in the context of the individual's overall presentation.

Nevertheless, the number of known risk factors present in any individual's personal circumstances must be taken into account in that person's risk management.

Table 1.5   Clinical risk indicators for suicide (adapted from Morgan, 2000).

Historical Previous self-harm Family history of suicide Previous use of violent methods	*Cognitive* Current suicidal thoughts/ideation Severe psychic anxiety Suicide plan Belief of no control over self/events
Physical Chronic physical illness/pain *Emotions* Hopelessness Helplessness	*Behaviour* Disengaged from services Poor adherence to psychiatric treatment Access/willingness to use lethal means
Diagnosis Depression Postnatal depression Alcohol and/or drug misuse Psychosis Puerperal psychosis	*Social* Unemployed/retired Separated/widowed/divorced Family concerned about risk Lack of social support
Verbal Expressed intent	*Other* Male gender Discharged from hospital within last 14 days

The suicidal crossroads?

Suicidal behaviour seems to increase when these factors converge:

1. Precipitating stressors occur in the recent *past*, e.g. the break up of a relationship, bereavement, loss of job etc.
2. These resonate with *more distant* stressors or traits that have hindered the development of the person's coping strategies and resilience as well as a 'rewriting' of the person's history that blots out most positive achievements and events.
3. The context of the *present* difficulties, e.g. the state of experiencing the situation as unbearable, feeling hopeless.
4. Greater hopelessness is a function of perceptions of the *future* which are lacking positivity, rather than filled with ideas of a negative future (Williams *et al.* 2005), with the individual:

a. literally unable to see positive outcomes and;
b. feeling trapped and unable to identify solutions to the problems they face (see Figure 1.4).

Feelings of hopelessness are highly correlated with suicide risk and it should be remembered that this is not always associated with depression. There are specific assessment scales that focus on hopelessness that can be useful but it is important to explore the extent and impact of this on the person's suicidal ideation.

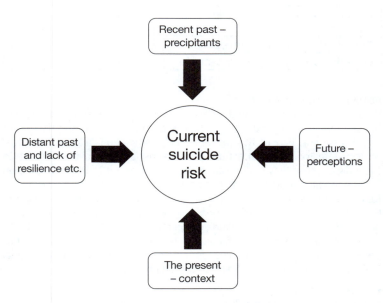

Figure 1.4   Factors affecting current suicide risk

Table 1.6   Groups with the highest risk of suicide (Eales 2006)

Group	Increased risk against the general population
Mental health patients within four weeks following discharge from hospital	× 100–200
People with a history of self-harm	× 10–30
People misusing drugs	× 10–20
People misusing alcohol	× 5–20
Offenders serving non-custodial sentences	× 8–13
Current or ex-mental health patients	× 10
Offenders serving a custodial sentence	× 9–10

Possible protective factors

Wherever possible, involving the person in identifying what might help her/him and what has reduced the risk before and why, are an essential part of any assessment. Part of this process is an examination of what individual protective factors might affect any potential risk(s). These will be unique to the individual but may be longstanding. It is important to try to develop an understanding not just of any protective factors but why these serve this function. Equally, you should explore what may impact upon that function. For example, someone with strong religious beliefs that have acted as a powerful deterrent to attempting suicide may well be at serious risk if s/he experiences a crisis of faith. Similarly, the loss of a relationship that has previously been very supportive and been a safeguard against suicidal feelings is likely to increase the risk. Possible protective factors may include:

- personal resilience;
- good problem-solving skills;
- future plans/hope for the future;
- strong religious faith or spiritual belief;
- belief that suicide is wrong;
- family responsibilities, e.g. as a carer;
- strong relationship with spouse/partner;
- strong social support;
- relationships and integration within community;
- economic security in older age;
- early identification and appropriate treatment of mental health problems (O'Brien and Hart 2013).

Twenty essential things to find out from the assessment of self-harm and/or suicide

1. Why now?
2. What were the precipitants?
3. What protective factors had prevented it until now?
4. What changed?
5. Were there specific mental health related issues, e.g. depression, command hallucinations?
6. Was the person influenced by anyone else's actions?
7. Was it premeditated or impulsive or spontaneous?
8. If it was premeditated, how much planning was involved?
9. Did the person provide any 'warnings' beforehand?
10. What stopped the attempt, e.g. did the person stop of her/his own volition or due to external causes?
11. Were the means used, e.g. tablets, acquired for this specific attempt?
12. What was the person's intention, e.g. to die, escape from an intolerable situation?
13. What did the person think might happen as a consequence of their attempt?
14. How did the person think other people might have responded?
15. Was the attempt itself controlled or was there a loss of control?
16. What did the person do after the attempt?
17. How was s/he found?
18. How does the person feel now they have survived?
19. Would they make a further attempt?
20. How does the person see their future?

Risk of dangerousness, violence and/or homicide

This is an area of clinical work that inevitably arouses high emotions both amongst clinicians and the public. Descriptive terms are often used inappropriately and in highly subjective ways, which can lead to misunderstanding, the labelling of people and unhelpful responses from staff (Repper and Perkins 2003).

Even referring to the literature, there are varying definitions of commonly used terms. Therefore the definitions offered below should be treated with caution. It is far better to actually describe the act that has taken place rather than using generic terms, e.g. 'Michael was shouting loudly, swearing and making threats to staff. He then threw a chair across the room at Staff Nurse Murray which narrowly missed her legs', or 'Michael shouted at Nurse Murray, saying that he would hit her if she did not leave the room but walked away without any intervention'. If generic terms such as 'anger' or 'violence' are used, the clinician should be as precise and accurate as possible when communicating with others, either orally or in documentation.

Key definitions

- **Homicide:** the killing of another human being, intentionally or accidentally, with or without justification. Criminal homicide occurs when a person purposely, knowingly, recklessly or negligently causes the death of another. Murder and manslaughter are both examples of criminal homicide.
- **Violence:** attempts to use force to violate, inflict physical damage or harm.
- **Aggression:** a hostile attitude and overt behaviour *intended* to inflict physical, psychological or emotional damage on another individual.
- **Predatory aggression:** stalking and perpetration of violence on another person.
- **Social aggression:** unprovoked aggression that is directed at members of the same species or group for purposes of establishing dominance.
- **Defensive aggression:** attacks delivered when an animal or person feels 'cornered' or trapped by a threatening aggressor. This is the type of aggression most commonly perpetrated against clinicians by patients and usually occurs when the person perceives s/he is at risk from staff or in an unsafe environment.
- **Anger:** a normal, subjective emotional state involving physiological arousal and *associated cognitions*. The emphasis on the associated cognitions is important, as the state of physiological arousal is similar to that which occurs when people describe themselves as feeling anxious. It is the cognitive association of the state of physiological arousal and potential actions, which is key and *may* lead to a violent response.
- **Hostility:** exhibiting enmity or opposition, to others, objects or ideas. It can also be described as a personality trait which reflects the interpretation of others' actions as harmful and can result in anger.

Homicide

- In the UK (population c. 60.5 million) the homicide rate is about 1.1 per 100,000.
- Following several decades of a steady increase in the number of homicides in the UK, there has been decline since 2004–05 (see Table 1.7).

Looking in more detail at the 2009–10 statistics (619 homicides):

- Two-thirds of homicide victims (68 per cent) were male.
- Around three-quarters of female victims knew the main suspect, compared with half (50 per cent) of male victims.
- Just over half of female victims aged 16 or over had been killed by their partner, ex-partner or lover (54 per cent, 94 offences).
- The most common method of killing for both male and females continues to be by sharp instrument. In 2009–10, as in each of the last eight years, male and female victims were both more likely to be killed by a sharp instrument than any other method.
- The second most common method for male murders involves hitting or kicking (113 homicides, or 27 per cent).
- The second most common method for females murder was strangulation or asphyxiation (41 homicides, or 21 per cent).
- There were 41 shooting homicide victims in 2009–10.
- In terms of re-offender rates, two homicide offences recorded in 2009–10 were committed by a suspect who had been convicted of a homicide on a previous occasion (Evans 2011).

Homicide and mentally disordered offenders

- There are approximately 52 patient homicides per year.
- There were 249 cases of homicide by current or recent patients occurring between April 1999 and December 2003. This accounted for 9 per cent of all homicides occurring in England Wales during this period.
- Data shows no clear evidence for either a rise or a fall in the number of homicides by people with mental illness.
- There has been a rise in the number of perpetrators subsequently judged to have been mentally ill at the time of the offence but a fall in the number of people found guilty of manslaughter on grounds of diminished responsibility, i.e. mental illness contributed to the offence (Appleby *et al.* 2006).

Table 1.7   United Kingdom homicide rates, 1959–2011

Year	Number of homicides
1959–60	262
1969–70	396
1979–80	549
1989–90	555
1999–2000	760
2000–01	792
2001–02	891
2002–03	1,048 (includes 172 attributed to Harold Shipman)
2003–04	853
2004–05	868
2005–06	765 (includes 54 victims of the July bombings in London)
2006–07	759
2007–08	753
2008–09	651
2009–10	619
2010–11	642 (includes 12 victims of Cumbria shootings)

Homicides, schizophrenia and personality disorders
- The number of homicides by people with schizophrenia is around 30 per year – this is 5 per cent of all homicides.
- Half the perpetrators with schizophrenia were current or recent patients.
- One-third had no previous contact with services.
- Approximately 10 homicides per year are committed by people with a personality disorder.

The prevalence of schizophrenia in the population is 1 per cent or less. Though the numbers are very small, the five-fold prevalence of all homicides by people with schizophrenia is an important finding that correlates with other studies that have highlighted the relationship between schizophrenia and violence, albeit one which is not as strong as that between substance misuse, alcohol or personality disorder with violence. This emphasises the need to actively treat psychotic symptoms when those are linked to the risk of violence (Maden 2007).

Key risk factors in patient homicide include:

1. Risk of dangerousness;
2. History of violence;
3. Non-attendance of appointments;
4. Non-compliance with treatment;
5. The presence of psychotic symptoms.

Nonetheless, even when those factors were present in the history of patients who went on to commit homicide, at final service contact:

- 88 per cent of people were assessed as no immediate or 'low risk';
- 1 per cent were assessed as being 'high risk' (Appleby *et al.* 2006).

The relationship between mental illness and violence
There is some evidence that the prevalence of violence of people diagnosed with schizophrenia is higher (8 per cent) than that in the general population (2 per cent), but with a far higher relationship between alcohol abuse and violence (24 per cent), and of those people drug dependent engaging in violent behaviour (34 per cent) (Swanson *et al.* 1997).

Whereas the United States Justice Department reported that people with a history of mental illness but not abusing drugs or alcohol were responsible for 4.3 per cent of homicides, that figure rose to 25 per cent where the homicide was that of a parent (Allnutt *et al.* 2010).

The significance of the presence of psychotic symptoms is fully discussed by Allnutt *et al.* (2010), where it is noted that the risk of violence increases in cases where the person's symptoms are not being treated, particularly if this is due to the patient refusing treatment. Violent offences are often linked to delusional beliefs.

The problem is most acutely experienced in inpatient units. Several UK studies have found the numbers of inpatients who have perpetrated violence to be as high as 28–32 per cent. Daffern *et al.* (2007: 18) noted that:

> Staff's refusal of requests or demands of activity are often perceived by patients as annoying, unfair, disrespectful, unjust, frustrating or irritating. Aggression towards staff and patients seems to be commonly preceded by frustration and often appeared to have a tension reducing quality.

Key clinical tip

Inpatient settings, by their very nature, are unstable and there is likely to be high levels of fluctuation in overall disturbance. Re-assessment of individual patients is required not just when observable change occurs in that person's behaviour or circumstances, but when factors in the ward environment occur which could destabilise them, no matter how previously stable they had been.

Table 1.8   Risk factors in aggression and/or violence (adapted from Morgan 2000).

Historical	Verbal
Previous incidents of violence Previous use of weapons Previous dangerous impulsive acts Previous admissions to secure settings Known personal trigger factors	Denial of previous dangerous acts Expressing intent to harm others Increased volume of speech Describing angry and/or uncontrollable feelings Making threats
Physical	Cognitive
Increased physical arousal Exaggerated reactions Invasion of body space Sexually inappropriate behaviour Facial tension	Ruminating on angry feelings and events Preoccupation with violent fantasy Suspicious and/or perceives threat from others
Emotions	Specific symptoms
Anger and/or hostility Frustration Suspicion	Violent command hallucinations Paranoid delusions about others Morbid jealousy Passivity

Other	*Mental health diagnosis*
Male gender, under 35 years of age	Psychosis
Major life events	Personality disorder
Unstable living arrangements	Dementia
Recent discontinuation of, or non-compliance with, medication	Organic brain injury
	Misuse of drugs and/or alcohol
Non-attendance of appointments	Autism/Asperger's syndrome plus complex needs

Developing a common language for assessing and communicating risk

There are significant differences in the various types of risk assessment you might undertake, for example:

- a triage assessment for the purpose of referring to a specialist team;
- an initial assessment of risk to determine a risk management plan;
- a re-assessment of someone where risk has previously been established.

There are inherent problems in using terminology such as 'short, medium or long term' etc., as these are subjective and open to interpretation. Ideally, it is better to think of risk in terms of whether it is immediate, i.e. likely to happen now, or in the future, in which case what would need to happen to make it more likely the risk would become imminent? Again, rather than describe risk in vague language such as 'low', 'medium' or 'high' (when, for instance does 'medium term' begin and end?), it is more useful to describe risk in terms of risk factors. These can be as follows:

Static
These are fixed, historical factors e.g. gender, family history of suicide, violence, previous hospital admissions, previous risk incidents. They are not anything that can be changed, therefore not something to 'treat' and do not provide a guide about whether or not risk has changed in the current context. However, these can provide a baseline or guide to how the person may behave in certain circumstances, e.g. will they make

threats or have they carried out actual acts of violence in the past? As such, you cannot afford to ignore them.

Stable

These are long-term factors, e.g. diagnosis of personality disorder or mental health problems. Of course, in many cases, diagnosis can change, either as the person becomes better known to clinicians or as new information comes to light through the assessment and treatment process. It then becomes important to re-evaluate issues of risk. These factors are not liable to fluctuate in a short space of time or be as vulnerable to change as dynamic factors.

Dynamic

These are present but fluctuate in duration and intensity, e.g. hopelessness, stress, treatment adherence, substance misuse or the opportunity to act in a dangerous way. It is important to consider these *measurable* factors in terms of treatment. Minimising the factors and their impact on the person and her/his behaviour is important.

Future

This involves trying to anticipate potential risk(s), particularly given knowledge of past risks.

The nature of different elements of the person's risk profile can then be identified more clearly and precisely, which can allow the clinician to think about the focus of immediate and longer-term risk management plans. For example:

> 'Last night, William took 30 paracetamol 500mg tablets with the intention of killing himself *(this will now be a static risk factor)*. He has been clinically depressed for several months *(stable risk factor)* but is now feeling hopeless, can see no future for himself and has disengaged from services *(dynamic risk factors)*. He currently still has plans to kill himself, using tablets, self poisoning or hanging, given the opportunity *(future risk factor)*.'

However, there may be a desire to use terminology such as 'low', 'medium' and 'high' risk (as may be the case, for instance, for non-mental health clinicians who have conducted a relatively brief assessment, or perhaps a triage in an A&E department, and want to communicate the urgency of the referral to the mental health team taking the referral). It is then essential that there are written definitions that clinicians can refer to and the understanding of which is widely shared and acknowledged (see Table 1.9).

One of the significant advantages of using recognised screening or risk assessment tools is that they provide a common language.

Table 1.9   An example of definitions of risk levels (adapted from Hart *et al.* 2009).

Low risk	Action required
A patient who has been fully assessed will be deemed to be 'low risk' if: • there are no significant mental health problems present; • there may have been some risk behaviours present, e.g. excessive drinking or substance abuse, superficial cutting, but these have not led to significant physical harm and there are sufficient protective factors to suggest this is unlikely to change; • s/he has no current plans to harm her/himself and/or others; • s/he is not vulnerable to self-neglect or exploitation by others; • it is not thought there will be any deterioration, in the foreseeable future, in her/his mental state or situation that would significantly change the levels of risk.	• No immediate action is required to address issues related to the patient's risk factors. • It may be helpful to look at alternative coping strategies with the patient. • The patient may benefit from health education/advice about potentially harmful behaviours, e.g. drinking and/or substance abuse. • The patient may be referred to primary care or voluntary sector services, where potentially harmful behaviours can be addressed with the patient if s/he wishes, but this would be on a routine basis. • In a ward setting, the patient would be preparing for imminent discharge.

Medium risk	Action required
A patient who has been fully assessed will be deemed to be 'medium risk' if one or more of the following are present: • mental health problems; • s/he may already have self-injured or harmed others but the injuries sustained were not life threatening; • s/he may have plans to harm her/himself and/or others but these are not immediate; • while the risk factors are not current, there is a probability they may become present in the absence of care and treatment; • s/he would be vulnerable to serious self-neglect or exploitation by others in foreseeable circumstances; • there is the possibility of deterioration in her/his mental state or situation that may significantly change the levels of risk if s/he is not in receipt of mental health care and treatment.	• All areas of risk must be clearly identified, with exacerbating and protective factors. • Attempts should be made to engage the patient in active treatment to address risk factors, beginning with agreeing a risk management plan, incorporating who will be doing what to help the patient remain safe. • Alternative coping strategies should be explored and expanded upon if necessary. • If a risk management plan is agreed, this should be fully documented and communicated to all clinicians (and others) who may have a role in assisting the patient to remain safe. • If the patient doesn't wish to engage in any risk management, nor commit her/himself to remain safe, decisions are required about how best to assist the patient, including whether or not a more restrictive environment is required and if there is a need for a Mental Health Act assessment. • If this is not pursued, the patient should be advised about options for getting further help.

Medium risk	Action required
	• Relevant clinicians should be kept informed of risk issues and patient views about participating in activities to keep her/himself safe. • In a ward setting, a safety care plan identifying the patient's risk issues and how s/he will manage those, with the help of the team, should be the basis of risk management. • If the patient is unwilling to engage in this, the risk should be re-defined as 'high'.
High risk	**Action required**
A patient who has been fully assessed will be deemed to be 'high risk' if one or more of the following are present: • significant mental health problems; • s/he has immediate plans to seriously harm or kill her/himself and/or seriously harm others; • there are significant risk factors which are current; • there is a likelihood these will increase in the absence of mental health care and treatment; • s/he could be vulnerable to serious self-neglect or exploitation by others;	• All areas of risk must be clearly identified, including exacerbating and protective factors. • Attempts should be made to immediately engage the patient in active treatment to address risk factors, beginning with agreeing a risk management plan, incorporating who will be doing what to help the patient remain safe. • Action plan required, addressing immediate risk factors, including an ongoing treatment and care package, communicated to all clinicians involved as well as any other relevant parties.

High risk	Action required
• there is a likelihood of deterioration in the person's mental state or situation that will significantly increase the levels of risk if s/he is not in receipt of mental health care and treatment.	• If patient is not willing to engage, a safety care plan should be imposed: a more restrictive setting should be considered if possible and a Mental Health Act assessment arranged for the earliest possible time.

Note: Patients newly admitted to a mental health service and/or not fully assessed should be regarded as medium to high risk in terms of risk management.

Key clinical tip

Terminology such as 'high', 'low', 'short', 'medium' and 'long' term can all be highly subjective and lead to misunderstanding and errors. Wherever they have to be used, a team should have clear definitions of what they mean and ensure clinicians using them understand their meaning.

References and select bibliography

Alderdice, J. *et al.* (2010) *Self-harm, Suicide and Risk: Helping People who Self-harm*. London: Royal College of Psychiatry.

Allnutt, S., O'Driscoll, C., Ogloff, J.R.P., Daffern, M. and Adams, J. (2010) *Clinical Risk Assessment and Management: A Practical Manual for Mental Health Clinicians.* Sydney, NSW: Justice Health.

American Foundation for Suicide Prevention (1997) 'Suicide in women', in *Suicide Facts*.

Appleby, L., Shaw, J., Kapur, N., Windfuhr, K., Ashton, A., Swinson, N. and While, D. (2006) *Avoidable Deaths: Five Year Report by the National Confidential Inquiry into Suicide and Homicide By People with Mental Illness*. Manchester: University of Manchester.

Bebbington, P., Cooper, C., Minot, S., Brugha, T.S., Jenkins, R., Metzer, H. and Dennis, M. (2009) 'Suicide attempts, gender and sexual abuse:

Data from the British psychiatric morbidity survey 2000', *American Journal of Psychiatry*, 166: 1135–40.

Bergen, H., Hawton, K., Waters, K., Cooper, J. and Kapur, N. (2010) 'Psychosocial assessment and repetition of self-harm: The significance of single and multiple repeat episode analyses', *Journal of Affective Disorders* 123: 95–101.

Bhugra, D. and Desai, M. (2002) 'Attempted suicide in South Asian women', *Advances in Psychiatric Treatment*, 8: 418–23.

Brezo, J., Paris, J., Vitaro, F., Hebert, M., Trembley, R.E. and Turecki, G. (2008) 'Predicting suicide attempts in young adults with histories of childhood abuse', *British Journal of Psychiatry*, 193: 134–39.

Callaghan, P. and Waldcock, H. (eds) (2006) *The Oxford Handbook of Mental Health Nursing*. Oxford: Oxford University Press.

Cooper, J., Kapur, N., Webb, R., Lawlor, M., Guthrie, E., Mackway-Jones, K. and Appleby, L. (2005) 'Suicide after deliberate self-harm: A 4-year cohort study', *American Journal of Psychiatry,* 162: 297–303.

Cutliffe, J. (2005) 'Assessing risk of suicide and self-harm', in Barker, P. (ed.) *Psychiatric and Mental Health Nursing: The Craft of Caring*. London: Hodder Arnold.

Daffern, M., Howells, K. and Ogloff, J.R.P. (2007) 'The interaction between individual characteristics and the function of aggression in forensic psychiatric inpatients', *Psychiatry, Psychology and Law*, 14: 17–25.

Dawson, J.M. and Langan, P.A. (1994) 'Murder in families', *US Department of Justice, Office of Justice Programs, Bureau of Justice Statistics*.

Department of Health (2002) *National Suicide Prevention Strategy for England: Annual Report on Progress*. London: DoH.

Eales, S. (2006) *Risk Assessment and Management Workbook*. London: City University.

Evans, L. (2011) 'Murder rate: the trends that solve the crime', *Guardian,* 20 January 2011.

Faulkner, A. (1997) *Briefing No. 1 – Suicide and Deliberate Self-Harm*. London: Mental Health Foundation.

Gelder, M., Mayou, R. and Cowen, P. (2001) *Shorter Oxford Textbook of Psychiatry*. Oxford: Oxford University Press.

Guthrie, E., Kapur, N., Mackway-Jones, K., Chew-Graham, C., Moorey, J., Mendel, E., Marino-Francis, F., Sanderson, S., Turpin, C., Boddy, G., Tomenson, B. and Patton, G.C. (2001) 'Randomised controlled trial of brief psychological intervention after deliberate self poisoning', *British Medical Journal*, 323(7305): 135–37.

Harris, C. and Barraclough, B. (1997) 'Suicide as an outcome for mental disorders', *British Journal of Psychiatry,* 170: 205–28.

Harrison, A. and Hart, C. (eds) (2006) *Mental Health Care for Nurses: Applying Mental Health Skills in the General Hospital*. Oxford: Blackwell.

Hart, C., Colley, R. and Harrison, A. (2009) *Risk Assessment Matrix: A Screening Tool for Assessing Risk in A&E Departments*. Kingston. Kingston University and St George's University of London.

Hawton, K. (2005) 'Psychosocial treatments following attempted suicide', in Hawton, K. (ed.) *Prevention and Treatment of Suicide: From Science to Practice*. Oxford: Oxford University Press.

Hawton, K. and James, A. (2005) 'Suicide and deliberate self-harm in young people', *British Medical Journal*, 330: 891–94.

Hawton, K., Casey, D., Bale, E. *et al.* (2007) *Deliberate Self-harm in Oxford*. Oxford: University of Oxford, Centre for Suicide Research.

Hjelmeland, H., Hawton, K., Nordvik, H., Bille-Brahe, U., De Leo, D., Fekete, S., Haring, C., Kerkhof, J.F.M., Lonnqvist, J., Michel, K., Renberg, E.S., Schmmidtke, A., Van Heeringen, K. and Wasserman, D. (2002) 'Why people engage in parasuicide: a cross-cultural study of intentions', *Suicide and Life-threatening Behavior*, 32: 380–93.

Horne, O. and Paul, S. (2008) *Understanding Self-harm*. London: SANE.

Horrocks, J. (2002) 'Self poisoning and self injury in adults', *Clinical Medicine*, 2: 509–12.

King, M., Semlyen, J., See Tai, S., Killaspy, H., Osbourn, D., Popelyuc, D. and Nazareth, I. (2008) *Mental Disorders, Suicide and Deliberate Self-Harm in Lesbian, Gay and Bisexual People*. London: National Mental Health Development Unit.

Maden, T. (2007) *Treating Violence: A Guide to Risk Management in Mental Health*. Oxford: Oxford Univeristy Press.

Mental Health Foundation (2006) *Statistics on Mental Health*. www.mentalhealth.org.uk

Morgan, S. (2000) *Clinical Risk Management: A Clinical Tool and Practitioner Manual*. London: The Sainsbury Centre for Mental Health.

National Institute for Clinical Excellence (2004) *Self-Harm: The Short-term Physical and Psychological Management and Secondary Prevention of Self-Harm in Primary and Secondary Care*, Clinical Guideline 16. London: NICE.

National Self-harm Network: www.nshn.co.uk

NHS Centre for Reviews and Dissemination (1998) *Deliberate Self-harm. Effective Health Care*, Volume 4, Number 6. University of York: NHS Centre for Reviews and Dissemination.

NHS Information Centre (2012) www.hscic.gov.uk

O'Brien, J. and Hart, C. (2013) *Clinical Risk Assessment and Risk Management*. London: South West London and St George's Mental Health NHS Trust.

O'Connor, R.C., Rasmussen, S. and Hawton, K. (2009a) 'Predicting deliberate self-harm in adolescents: a six month prospective study', *Suicide and Life-Threatening Behavior*, 39: 364–75.

Office for National Statistics (2007) *Mortality Statistics*, Series DH2 no.s 30, 32.

Repper, J. and Perkins, R. (2003) *Social Inclusion and Recovery: A Model for Mental Health Practice*. London: Bailliere Tindall.

Royal College of Psychiatrists (2006) *Self-harm*. London: RCP.

Royal College of Psychiatrists (2008) 'Rethinking risk to others in mental health services', *Final Report of the Scoping Group*. London: RCP.

Smith, K. and Flatley, J. (eds) (2010) *Homicides, Firearm Offences and Intimate Violence 2008/09.* London: Home Office.

Swanson, J. W., Estroff, S., Swartz, M., Borum, R., Lachiotte, W., Zimmer, C. and Wagner, R. (1997) 'Violence and severe mental disorder in clinical and community populations: The effects of psychotic symptoms, comorbidity, and lack of treatment', *Psychiatry*, 60: 1–22.

Thomson, F., Sherring, S. and Garnham, P. (2010) *A Guide to the Assessment and Management of Risk.* London: Oxleas NHS Foundation Trust.

Williams, J.M.G., Crane, C., Barnhofer, T. and Duggan, D. (2005) 'Psychology and suicidal behaviour: elaborating the entrapment model', in Hawton, K. (ed.) *Prevention and Treatment of Suicidal Behaviour: From Science to Practice.* Oxford: Oxford University Press.

Zahl, D. and Hawton, K. (2004) 'Repetition of deliberate self-harm and subsequent suicide risk: long-term follow-up study in 11,583 patients', *British Journal of Psychiatry,* 185: 70–75.

Part 2: General principles of risk assessment

This section of the *Pocket Guide* identifies specific approaches to risk assessment and management, issues to consider before, during and after assessment and assessment techniques.

Identifying risks, or picking out risk factors, only provides the information about risk to then be assessed. That is completed when the likelihood and consequences of the person acting have been worked through and leads to the risk management plan.

Although there will be occasions when assessments need to be undertaken over an extended period, most risk assessments – as opposed to a comprehensive mental health assessment – can be conducted in a relatively brief period of time by staff who have received appropriate education and training, even if they do not work in a mental health setting.

For example, A&E department nurses can conduct a mental health triage, incorporating a risk assessment, in 15 to 20 minutes with sufficient competence to make an accurate referral to specialist mental health teams. Similarly, paramedics who have been trained in the process and structure of risk assessment can conduct a risk assessment and develop a risk management plan, referring to the appropriate agency, even if that is simply to ensure the patient is taken to the nearest A&E department for further assessment and treatment.

General Practitioners and senior clinicians in primary care can do the same. Again, this is predicated on them having received sufficient training from mental health experts, having a triage or assessment framework, and access to expert advice and clinical supervision. Of course, many GPs and others in primary care have great experience in this area and assess and work in the community with people trying to cope with significant risks before making referrals to specialist mental health services.

Different approaches to risk assessment

There are a number of approaches to risk assessment. However, there is a lot of evidence that the most effective is the structured professional judgement, or structured clinical assessment (see below). Other approaches are mentioned in passing only so readers can consider which they currently use and their rationale for doing so.

Structured professional judgement, or structured clinical assessment

This is not a specific assessment instrument but combines:

- the evidence base for risk factors;
- an individual, structured patient assessment;
- a formulation;
- a risk management plan (Bouch and Marshall 2005).

Using this approach your decision is informed by aspects of an actuarial approach and background information. However, the application of clinical judgement is also required, demonstrating:

- the ability to weigh up the information gained through the assessment itself against any clinical risk factors identified;
- integrating this within any algorithms prescribed by your organisation;
- using this combination of tools and information to come to a reasoned decision that addresses the key issues in the patient's situation.

The unstructured clinical approach

This is based on the clinicians' judgement alone, consequent to her/his assessment and without reference to assessment tools or clinical risk indicators, etc. It is thus dependent on the clinician's experience and highly subjective and, therefore, not recommended (Bouch and Marshall 2005; Maden 2007).

The actuarial approach

This stems from compiling and analysing statistics in the world of insurance for the purposes of calculating risks and, therefore, premiums. Forensic psychiatry first adapted this methodology to try and predict dangerousness and risk. It involves:

- formal assessment methods such as the use of assessment tools, e.g. the HCR-20;
- the use of clinical algorithms or protocols.

The actuarial approach follows 'objective' procedures to classify risk, looking at probability and predictability. For example, clinical algorithms are 'an explicit description of appropriate steps to be taken in the care of a patient with a particular problem', which should account for a full clinical history, with subsequent recommendations for diagnosis and/or treatment based on the data obtained. Algorithms include 'branching logic', which allows recommendations to be 'individualised according to the patient's age, gender and specific clinical findings' (Komaroff 1982).

Of course, assessing the likelihood of dangerous behaviour in the context of mental health problems is not the same as assessing chest pain or simply basing a prediction of future behaviour on what has gone before. It involves a degree of clinical assessment and this should be taken into account when considering the reliability of using an actuarial approach, which is of very limited value on its own (Bouch and Marshall 2005).

Making use of the information gained from assessment

The wider the sources of your information, the more opportunity there is to deliberate on potential risks. However, the absence of information must not be a barrier to making decisions when they are urgently required, and clinicians need to be mindful that they are not pursuing information that will be either irrelevant or over-complicate the decision-making process. Key factors include:

- accessing documented information and records about the individual's own history, particularly in relation to previous risk behaviours. This is best done in their original form wherever possible, rather than through second-hand reports, e.g. looking at a contemporary account of a hospital admission rather than a subsequent reference to it in a later summary;
- exploring the individual's current situation, mental state and behaviour in the context of clinical risk indicators (see Table 2.1);

- a comprehensive interview aimed at gaining information about the person – it is important to note the difference between a face-to-face assessment and the significant limitations placed upon the clinician conducting a telephone triage or assessment;
- obtaining corroborating information from those who know the patient, e.g. family members, carers, the GP, other health and social care professionals and other agencies such as the police;
- the use of rating scales.

Determining the risk will then occur in the context of:

- your judgements based on this information;
- knowledge of risk indicators and how they relate to your assessment;
- your reaction, based on your experience and sense of the person, often, incorrectly, referred to as 'intuition' or 'gut feeling' but tapping into what Aristotle termed 'phronesis', the knowledge assimilated through the process of experience, in this case repeated clinical assessments – see also Gladwell (2005) for an interesting discussion on this issue.

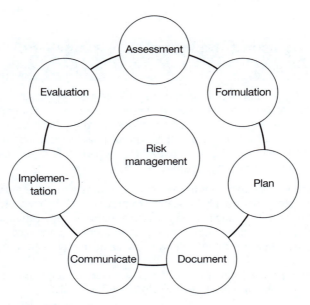

Figure 2.1 The formula for risk management

Translating the assessment into a formulation

Any assessment has to be accompanied by a formulation, i.e. a concept-ualisation of:

1. What has happened;
2. Who is affected by the event(s);
3. How it has happened;
4. Where it happened;
5. Why it has happened.

(See the 'Developing a formulation' section in Part 3, page 129.)

Use the **FACT** principles in risk assessment:

Fast
Accurate
Comprehensive
Therapeutic

The safety of the clinician and patient

Table 2.1 Safety and the referral process.

Is the purpose of the referral clear?
Is it clear what the team are being asked to assess?
Have any known risks been clearly identified?
Is more information required?
Who should undertake the assessment – and why?
Ideally, where should the assessment take place?
How urgent is it?
Note: All first assessments outside of a clinical setting, e.g. a health centre and, for example, in the patient's home, should be undertaken by two people (see below).

Crucial to risk assessment is the safety of the clinician. Consideration of this begins from the moment information is being gathered through to the referral process (see below). The referral should initially be reviewed by the clinical team wherever possible and a strategy devised to address any known or potential risks.

The next issue to consider is whether or not the environment is a safe one in which the assessment can take place. Issues discussed in other sections will also impact upon safety, e.g. the clinician's ability to 'contain' the patient's anxiety and distress/disturbance, as well as the ability to minimise the patient's level of arousal.

Key clinical tip

Under no circumstances should clinicians compromise their own safety. Take every opportunity to make the assessment process safe for yourself and it will be safer for the patient.

If in the patient's home

Even before visiting the person's home, risk can be weighed:

- Is it safe for one person to visit on her/his own?
- Is the surrounding area safe?
- If you are visiting by car, can it be parked to allow an easy and swift exit?
- What are the entrances/exits like? Can access and, particularly, egress be easily blocked?
- If the patient lives in a block of flats, what risks are there in the general environment?
- Do team members know exactly where you are, i.e. the patient's address?
- Have you informed them of the time you are entering the premises and time you plan to finish?
- Check that you have adequate reception for your mobile phone before entering.
- By this time, before you enter, you will have effectively conducted a necessary 'doorstep assessment', which will determine whether or not you enter and conduct your full assessment.

Key clinical tip

If you have serious concerns about your safety do not enter the premises. If you begin to have concerns once you are in, provide a pre-prepared reason and leave immediately.

When entering the premises

- Follow the person in rather than allowing them to remain by the door while you go in first.
- Check the environment for potential weapons, while taking account of the likelihood they might be used. It is worth noting that, in someone's home, the kitchen is obviously a place where there are a lot of potentially dangerous things that could be used as weapons, e.g. knives. In other rooms, there will be any number of commonplace items that could be dangerous but the key issue is how potentially dangerous you view the person you are assessing and whether or not there are any obvious weapons visible.
- Are there any others on the premises who might pose a potential risk? For example, you might know a particular family member has a history of violence. Equally, there may be people you know nothing about, and weren't expecting to be there, in another room, while general activity in the accommodation, such as drug taking, might be a cause for concern.
- Take a seat nearest the exit.
- Be mindful about discussing issues that lead to the patient becoming highly aroused beyond the point where you feel confident s/he can contain her/himself or you can de-escalate the situation.
- Leave if the situation changes and you have serious doubts about your safety.
- Have a 'codeword' arranged with your team that can be used in an innocuous phrase, signalling you require immediate assistance. If you sense you are in potential danger and tell the patient you need to make a phone call telling someone you will be delayed, this would allow you to use the word, e.g. it might be Osbourne, so saying, 'Please contact Mr Osbourne to let him know I'm running late…' will alert your colleagues that you need assistance.
- Have your mobile phone switched to speed dial for ready assistance.

- If you have concerns about the safety of the visit but have decided, on balance, to proceed with it, agree a time with the team by which you will have checked in with them, either in person, or by phone.

If on a ward or inpatient unit/outpatient department

- Decide who should carry out the assessment and how many staff should be involved in the actual assessment.
- Have staff available for support if needed, having decided where they should be positioned, e.g. out of sight, outside the room, in the room etc.
- Ensure colleagues know:
    - any potential risks;
    - where you are;
    - what you're doing;
    - how long you will be;
- Sit nearest the exit and within reach of alarm buttons.
- Place the chairs so they are a comfortable distance from one another and at an angle, which means you are not directly facing the patient but can easily establish eye contact (check to see if the patient is comfortable with the configuration).
- Minimise the potential for interruptions.

Taking a referral

This involves the gathering of as much information in advance of the assessment as possible, with an emphasis on the following:

- Any known specifics about risk: current, in the past and potential. If there is unsubstantiated speculation about possible risk, this should also be considered.
- If a previous risk assessment has been carried out and is available to the referrer, you should expect to receive a copy in advance of seeing the patient. However, this should not be thought to exclude the need to do a new risk assessment or even a full assessment, remembering context and circumstances are different and the person's internal view of their past and personal history may have changed.
- What, exactly, the referrer sees as the purpose of the referral and any action they expect to be taken, as well as any future involvement they would expect to have.

However, it is equally important that the referral process is straightforward for referrers, with no barriers. For example, arbitrary definitions of 'crisis' or referral criteria that do not match service need may create delays, confusion and further problems and become significant risk factors in themselves.

The referrer's perception of the urgency or immediacy of the referral has to be acknowledged and addressed, with appropriate levels of support and assistance offered to help them and the patient, whether or not the person will be seen as quickly as the referrer initially thinks necessary. Assisting the referrer in understanding available resources and what they can do to address the situation prior to the patient being seen is an important part of the process.

Ongoing dialogue about referrals and how they will be treated can help educate referrers and improve the standard, quality and appropriateness of referrals.

Use the STAR principles in taking a referral

The referral process should be:

Simple
Transparent
Accessible
Rapid

Gathering information

The patient should be regarded as the relevant expert in her/his life and the principal source of any information, which can be gained through a face-to-face interview. The importance of this is not just in conversation but direct observation, noting the congruence of what is said, tone of voice, body language and posture. When discussing attitudes and feelings, it has been estimated that only 7 per cent is communicated through the content of *what* is actually said, with 38 per cent arising from *how* it is said, e.g. tone of voice, and the final 55 per cent through body language, e.g. facial expression, gestures, posture and body movement (Mehrabian 1981).

Though the amount of communication through body language will vary when different themes are being communicated, the ability to see the person providing the information is obviously crucial when assessing serious risk. For example, there will be gestures and non-verbal acts that illustrate or emphasise particular points the person is talking about; affect displays or facial configurations will reveal emotional states that may be related or unrelated to the topic of discussion and are often unconscious. Gestures associated with this are often spontaneous and can be a better guide to how the person is feeling than what they are saying (Hannagan 2007).

Working with families/carers and issues of confidentiality

Further information and corroboration should be gained from patient records, family members, carers, and health, social care or other professionals who have had contact with the patient.

Permission should be sought from the person before seeking information from other sources but, if there are serious concerns about the safety of the individual or others, these should outweigh issues of confidentiality and it is important to obtain the information even if the individual hasn't agreed.

Even with the greater emphasis on confidentiality in recent years, it must always be remembered that communicating serious concerns with other healthcare professionals and/or agencies about the safety of an individual and/or the public will supersede requirements about confidentiality.

Working constructively with carers and families is an essential part of the risk assessment and risk management process.[1] If families or friends are concerned that someone may be at risk, it is important that they are able to voice their concerns and that these will be fully considered during the assessment process. As already noted, it has been widely recognised in many serious inquiries that carer and family concerns were not given sufficient credibility, nor warnings from them heeded by clinical teams.

Equally, they should be given information and support as soon as possible. Even when it is clear there are significant risk issues, family or friends may fear saying the wrong thing. It is useful for you to establish as early as possible what information, if any, the patient is willing to share with relatives and/or carers (O'Brien and Hart 2013). However, supporting families by providing general advice does not break confidentiality, as is shown in the examples below:

Example 1: *'I can't speak to you about your daughter without her permission, but I can tell you if someone has a condition such as you've described, these are the symptoms to look out for…'*

Example 2: *'If you're worried about someone experiencing this, or maybe beginning to experience this, then please call the team on this number…'*

Key clinical tip

In many suicide and homicide inquiries, it has emerged that the concerns of family members and/or carers were not given sufficient importance. Their input should be a key consideration in your assessment.

References and selected bibliography

Bouch, J. and Marshall, J.J. (2005) 'Suicide risk: structured professional judgement', *Advances in Psychiatric Treatment,* 11: 84–91.

Department of Health (2011) *Consultation on Preventing Suicide in England: A Cross-government Outcomes Strategy to Save Lives.* London: DoH.

Gladwell, M. (2005) *Blink: The Power of Thinking Without Thinking.* London: Penguin.

Goleman, D. (1996) *Working with Emotional Intelligence.* London: Bloomsbury.

Hannagan, T. (2007) *Management,* 5th edition. London: Prentice Hall.

Harrison, A. (2006) 'Self-harm and suicide prevention', in Harrison, A. and Hart, C. (eds) *Mental Health Care for Nurses: Applying Mental Health Skills in the General Hospital.* Oxford: Blackwell.

Hawton, K., Harriss, L. and Zahl, D. (2006) 'Deaths from all causes in a long term follow up study of 11,583 deliberate self harm patients', *Psychological Medicine,* 36: 397–405.

Komaroff, A.L. (1982) 'Algorithms and the 'art' of medicine', *American Journal of Public Health,* 72(1): 10–12.

Maden, T. (2007) *Treating Violence: A Guide to Risk Management in Mental Health.* Oxford: Oxford University Press.

Mehrabian, A. (1981) *Silent Messages: Implicit Communication of Emotions and Attitudes,* 2nd edition. Belmont, California: Wadsworth.

Morgan, S. and Wetherell, A. (2009) 'Assessing and managing risk', in Norman, I. and Ryrie, I. (eds) *The Art and Science of Mental Health Nursing*, 2nd edition. Berkshire: Open University Press.

O'Brien, J. and Hart, C. (2013) *Clinical Risk Assessment and Risk Management.* London: South West London and St George's Mental Health NHS Trust.

Note

1 Family members are often the main carers. If carers and/or family members have a role in any risk management plan, it is important that they have agreed to this and their role is clear to everyone, including the patient. This should be documented in the risk management plan and all relevant parties should have a copy of this plan. You need to remember also that family members may be at an increased risk in some instances against members of the general public and this needs to be incorporated into any risk management strategy.

Part 3: Undertaking a risk assessment

First impressions

Having established a safe environment and provided the person being assessed with sufficient information about the process, the formal part of the assessment starts. An important issue arises from your very first impression on seeing the person. This may be as you walk into the reception area of a health centre, a room on a ward or into the person's home.

The whole thrust of texts about risk assessment is about careful, nuanced, in-depth analysis and decision-making. Yet, first impressions often create an instant reaction and, whether or not we welcome them, can have a powerful impact on our judgement (Gladwell 2005). Are these trustworthy? Research undertaken into the adaptive unconscious strongly suggests there is evidence that first impressions can tell us a lot about someone and/or a situation (and there is even richer 'information' when the first meeting is in the person's home).

The kind of observations that might be useful include:

- What do you see?
- What is the person's facial expression and demeanour?
- What, specifically, did you notice?
- What were they doing at the moment you saw them?
- Did they make eye contact or look away?
- Did they change their posture and, if so, in what way?
- Did the person meet your expectations – and what were those expectations?
- How did you feel, and what was it about the person that led you to feel like that? For example, if you're suddenly feeling anxious, what has caused that?
- Most importantly, was that first impression borne out by what you learned about the person during the rest of the assessment?
- If not, what was different?

It is important to remember that this initial impression might tap into unconscious negative attitudes or even prejudices, e.g. about 'people who self-harm' and might influence the interaction without the clinician being aware. The clinician may also 'follow' her/his apparent instinct about the patient, seeking information that reinforces it and not looking to establish as broad a picture as might otherwise have been the case.

However, self-awareness about one's own potential negative attitudes can help counterbalance these risks. Practice – the act of doing a number of assessments and risk assessments, building from being supervised to either undertaking them alone or leading in the process but doing them frequently and regularly – assists in the development of what Aristotle termed *phronesis*, usually translated as practical wisdom or prudence. Aristotle noted that certain types of knowledge can only become known through experience rather than teaching or formal learning. It has also been termed innominate knowledge. This has been described as knowledge that is derived from practice, experience, doing things over and over, rather than theory or organised study. It is what is often – wrongly – termed 'intuition'. This is the type of rapid decision-making that experienced people in many different walks of life exercise, apparently 'on a hunch' or 'gut feeling' but which is actually more likely the result of having gone through the same process so many times that every nuance and the many small signs that might not be recognisable by a less experienced practitioner are recognisable, where the incongruence of someone's body language or facial expression with their verbal response immediately rings alarm bells or satisfies the clinician that what s/he is hearing is likely to be an accurate reflection of how the person is actually feeling and thinking.

Key clinical tip

Make a careful mental note of your first impression, while being mindful of any potential prejudices.

Initial communications and developing a rapport

It is important not to assume you have a willing partner in the assessment. Gauging the patient's degree of collaboration must be integral in determining the risk. However, this is not a static process. The way in which the clinician builds and develops a rapport and seeks the individual's collaboration and agreement in the assessment process is crucial to how the risks change. Feeling comfortable and engaged in the process is likely to help the person talk more freely about their experiences and seek helpful solutions while interpersonal problems experienced in the early stages of an interview will undoubtedly complicate the process and make it more difficult.

Helping the patient understand the purpose of the interview and how it will be conducted will assist in developing a rapport (see Table 3.1). A collaborative process also involves the clinician 'entering the world' of the patient, however 'disturbed' this might be, embracing the person's current experience of the world and exploring this without judgement or prejudice. An empathic acceptance of the patient's experience and communicating that their responses can be understood and make sense within the context of their background and/or current circumstances can be invaluable (Linehan 1993).

How does this work in practice? It may be very difficult to understand someone talking about a conspiracy theory, plots to harm him and

Table 3.1 Information to provide to the patient at the start of the assessment

The purpose and nature of the interview.
Approximately how long it will take/how much time you have available.
You will be asking a number of potentially 'difficult' questions – and the rationale for doing so.
Questions don't have to be answered but it is helpful to do so.
There will be an opportunity for the patient to ask questions.
What will happen with the information provided.
What happens next.

unseen forces at work to do things he believes place him in serious danger. However, without colluding with delusional beliefs, to be curious about this world, to want to understand how it works, how the person makes sense of what is happening and how they *feel* as a consequence, as well as what they have decided to do because of what is 'happening', doesn't just validate their experience but provides invaluable information for the clinician.

It should be remembered that if the person is compliant simply because they fear a more coercive response from the clinician should they be obviously resistant, e.g. detention under the Mental Health Act, this is *not* concordance and interventions should be gauged accordingly (see Figure 3.1). Identifying reasons for non-compliance, if present, are as important as anything else in the assessment and make any response and attempt to improve collaboration more effective. Reasons could include:

- lack of insight or disagreeing with the wider understanding and interpretation of the person's mental state, behaviour or view of the world;
- denial or minimisation of the problem;
- guilt;
- a desire to maintain control and independence.

While it is important to seek permission as part of the collaborative process, and offer the individual the option of not answering questions that cause distress or are uncomfortable, you need to think through how to try and access information the person is unwilling or finding difficult to impart. For example:

- Have you asked too probing a question too early?
- Does the person understand what you mean?
- Could you have phrased the question better?
- Does the person feel too embarrassed to answer?
- Is it too distressing to answer?
- Is the person being evasive?
- Is s/he unwilling to cooperate with you?

There is a possibility that, if you are unable to obtain the information to enable you to make a reasoned judgement and decision with the person about managing the risk, you will need to consider more restrictive options.

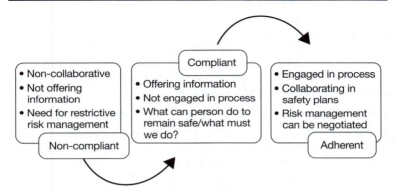

Figure 3.1 The relationship between the degree of collaboration and the risk management plan

---

Key clinical tip

Good communications skills help develop a rapport. Using this rapport from the outset allows you to help the person tell their story and can promote thinking about solutions even while taking an apparently problem-dominated history.

Establishing a rapport – skills needed

Whether sitting down in a clinical situation with an individual you haven't met before or meeting someone who is well known to you through your clinical practice, you should be thinking of either building or maintaining a 'therapeutic relationship' with that person.

As noted by Reynolds (2003: 139), 'the therapeutic relationship is not a nebulous, kind hearted, well intentioned relationship'. For the purposes of this *Pocket Guide*, there is no need to go into great detail but it is worth thinking about how this enables the risk assessment to proceed as easily as possible. Stuart (2005: 15) defines it as, '[a] mutual learning experience and a corrective emotional experience for the patient'. The clinician will use 'personal attributes and clinical techniques in working with the patient' to 'enable her/him to learn more satisfactory and productive patterns of behaviour' (Reynolds 2003: 140).

An early stage of building any new relationship, often termed the orientation phase, is to develop a *rapport*. It is important to distinguish between the skills required for building a rapport with someone you don't know, for what is likely to be a 'one-off' contact, from those used to develop a therapeutic relationship over the longer term, as there are subtle differences to the skills and process.

Building a rapport involves skills familiar to most healthcare staff:

• Looking for common ground – the most important aspect of this is the way in which the clinician focuses on the person being assessed, using the techniques outlined below. It can also mean picking up on 'small things', such as shared interests, commenting on aspects of the person's experience and story that are not necessarily clinically relevant. However, one thing that should almost always be shared is the desire to find a solution to the current 'problem' or reason the person is with you at that moment, as well as then helping that person 'move on'. Of course, there may well be disagreement about how, and how quickly, that will happen. Nonetheless, to make this a stated purpose of the assessment can often be helpful (and it may not be clear to the person being assessed unless explicitly said), after which the clinician's negotiating skills may well be required to give it genuine meaning for the person.
• Courtesy and respect for the person, sometimes despite her/his behaviours.
• Interest in the person's story.
• Empathy.
• Building trust by:
    – being honest
    – being clear about the purpose of the contact
    – being genuine
    – giving information.

However, it also involves some skills that we might use but not necessarily knowingly:

Pacing
This means 'entering' the other person's world by:

• listening to and observing the other person carefully;
• reflecting what he or she knows and regards as important and true and matching some part of their ongoing experience.

We can pace a person's mood, body language and speech patterns, including tone, volume, and the type of words, phrases and images that person uses. You can even pace their breathing patterns as a way of building a rapport. You obviously do not want to be as loud or physically active as someone who is very aroused and behaving in a disturbed or distressed manner; nor would you want to be as slowed down and psychologically retarded as a depressed person. However, pacing allows you to gradually exert influence over the other person, either by slowing down the communication with the aroused person or subtly lifting the depressed person, bringing them to your pace.

Mirroring

This involves getting into rhythm with the person on as many levels as possible, e.g. talking in the way that s/he talks, sitting the way that s/he sits, moving in the general patterns that he or she is moving.

Clinical example 1: Giving information and developing a rapport

Clinician: Hello, William, as I said earlier, my name is John. This is my colleague, Jenny, and we're from the Community Mental Health Team. We're based at the local mental health centre and we see everyone referred to us from this area. Thanks very much for letting us come and see you.

William: Yeah, well, I'm still not sure what you're here for.

Clinician: As I wrote in my letter, we've been asked by your GP...

William: [*Interrupts*] I saw that. But why does she want me to see you? What's it all for?

Clinician: She wanted us to come and see you because, as I understand it, you'd told her you were having trouble sleeping and have been having panic attacks and some other experiences that you'd found worrying. Is that right?

William: Yeah, but I told her I'd be okay and then she said I needed to see you lot again.

Clinician: It sounds as if you were reluctant to see us?

William: Absolutely. I didn't want to see you. And I told her that.

Clinician: But those worries about not sleeping and the panic attacks were serious enough at the time for you to seek help?

William: [Pause]. Yes … and that's why I wanted some sleeping tablets, because I'm up all night and that was driving me nuts, same as the funny turns.

Clinician: Are you still up all night and having funny turns?

William: Yes. But I don't … I don't want to have to see anyone about it.

Clinician: What particularly is worrying you about seeing us today?

William: I don't want to end up back in hospital. And I've got the dog now. I couldn't leave her.

Clinician: I've got a dog, They can be a worry, even though they're great fun. She's a little like yours but a bit smaller. Yours has a lovely temperament. Is she good company?

William: Yes.

Clinician: Mine's the same, but not as friendly as yours. But, back to you… You're worried if you talk to us, you might end up in hospital?

William: I did last time.

Clinician: Obviously, neither Jenny or I knew you then but I've had a chance to read your notes and I did see you were unhappy about being in hospital then, so I'm not that surprised you're reluctant to talk to us today. But I've spoken to Dr Jones and she didn't think she had the particular skills to really help you just now. She said she was very worried things were getting on top of you.

William: She said that?

Clinician: Yes. Which is why she got in touch with us. I'm happy to go at your pace. I thought we might look at ways in which we could help you prevent things getting any worse, like helping you get some sleep, and doing something about those funny turns, as well as talking about what's been happening recently.

William: I'm not sure I'm ready for that.

Clinician: Well, as I said, we can go at your pace. And it can't be a nice feeling to think you're going nuts in the middle of the night.

William: It isn't.

> **Key clinical tip**
>
> You have to work to develop a rapport. Be attentive, mindful and ready to enter the person's 'world' and try to understand her/his perspective without colluding or saying things you don't believe to be true.

Non-verbal communication

So much that's written about assessment focuses on what is said, yet as we have noted, most of our communication is non-verbal. As we need to focus attention on the non-verbal communication of the patient, we also have to be mindful not only of what we are communicating without speaking but also how our body language, posture and physical presence can be used to assist the assessment process.

We should remember that most people being interviewed are likely to be experiencing some degree of anxiety, if not directly as a consequence of their mental state then in relation to being 'assessed', which they may equate with being 'judged', or having possible negative outcomes.

It can, therefore, be 'containing', psychologically, for the person being interviewed if you are able to present yourself in a calm, thoughtful and open manner, be able to listen without judgemental comments or responses and set boundaries where required while being flexible enough to respond to the individual's needs (see Table 3.2).

Always consider whether or not your **body language**, **facial expression** and **tone of voice** are congruent with what you are saying. If they're not, you need to consider why that might be the case:

- How are you feeling towards the patient?
- Is there something going on in the interview that you are finding difficult or feel uncomfortable about?
- Might it be something you 'brought in' with you from a previous session or outside work?
- How are you going to deal with it in the assessment, while you're with the patient?

Table 3.2 Putting the person at ease with your non-verbal communication and physical presence.

Seating	Place the chairs you will use comfortably angled at approximately 90 degrees (when possible), so both people can make eye contact but not be looking directly at one another. Barriers, such as a table, should be removed if possible. It is also useful to simply ask the patient if s/he is comfortable with the seating arrangement – though you should always remember to place yourself in the chair with the easiest access to the exit and alarm buttons. That is not negotiable.
Maintain eye contact	Even if the patient does not meet your gaze, continue to look at her/him. It both aids your own assessment of the person but, when s/he looks back at you, will indicate your continued interest if your gaze is still there to be met.
Build confidence and a sense of safety	Physically communicate your own *confidence* and sense of *safety* by appearing calm, by thinking about the situation and remaining engaged in the person's story, no matter how distressing.
Be patient	Allow the patient time to answer your questions.

Key interview skills

There are a wide range of techniques that are going to be used in specific parts of an assessment. However, key aspects that will be used throughout, which are often a mix of verbal and non-verbal skills, will be useful in helping the person express difficult feelings and tackle difficult issues with you (see Box 5 below).

Box 5: Key interview skills

- Having an interview structure with which you are familiar. It allows you to follow the person's story and facilitate digression if necessary but return to the important issues you need to explore.
- Employing active listening – communicate to the patient that you are both listening and interested in her/his story.
- Demonstrating empathy .
- Looking for non-verbal cues:
  - Is there congruence between body language, facial expression and dialogue?
  - Does the person want you to pursue a line of inquiry?
  - Is s/he reluctant to answer a particular question?
  - Is s/he angry, sad, distressed?
  - Does s/he understand what you're saying?
  - If there is silence is it because s/he's not willing to respond, reflecting on what's been said already or is s/he thinking of what to say?
- Providing 'containment'.

Demonstrating empathy

Empathy is a complex, multi-dimensional response and cannot be 'acted'. It involves cognition, emotions and behaviour but also requires a focus on the other person through the careful use of observation.

Active, or reflective, listening leads to a cognitive process of reasoning and understanding, which in turn then has to be conveyed to the person to whom you are listening. This can be done in a variety of ways – for example:

- Seeking to explore and clarify feelings, e.g. 'How did you feel about your father's death?'
- Responding to feelings, e.g. 'I'm sorry to hear that. It sounds as if it was very upsetting for you.'
- Exploring the personal meaning of feelings, e.g. 'Were you upset about your own loss or was it because of the painful way in which he died?'

Given that many people find it difficult to articulate their emotions, the ability to 'read' non-verbal cues such as body language, gestures, facial expression and tone of voice are key to intuiting others' emotions. It should come as no surprise then that nodding, the use of facial expression, pacing and mirroring will also demonstrate empathy. There is also evidence from exercises in studying the ability to 'read' others' expressions and non-verbal cues which has demonstrated that these are skills that can be learned through experience and exposure (Goleman 1996).

Containing the person's anxiety during the assessment

Containment is a very difficult concept to both grasp and practise but is simply defined by Casement (1985) as, responding to '[t]imes when people can't cope with their own feelings without assistance' and that the assistance being sought is 'for a person to be available to help with these difficult feelings' [emphasis in the original]. Casement also likens this process to:

- 'holding' the person in a psychological rather than physical sense;
- being available;
- offering understanding and, where appropriate, insight;
- perhaps most importantly, being able to facilitate the person to talk about and then tolerate the feelings they find most difficult.

Clinical example 2: Containing the person's anxiety

William: I can't talk about that.

Clinician: Can you tell me what makes it so difficult?

William: It's just too awful.

Clinician: I get the sense that you think about this thing a lot, whatever it is, so I'm not sure what would be different in talking about it. Do you worry it might be too much for me?

William: Why would anyone want to hear about my mess?

Clinician: Is that part of the reason you tried to kill yourself?

William: [Long silence] Yes. In part.

Clinician: Is there anything that might make it easier to talk about your feelings?

William:	What, talk about how I couldn't wait for my Dad to die, that all the time he was suffering I didn't really care, I just wanted it over?
Clinician:	Is it true you didn't care?
William:	It was just too much.
Clinician:	So, was it that you simply wanted him to die, or that you felt overwhelmed to see him suffer so much?

In this example, the clinician does not labour the point about it being difficult for the patient to articulate his feelings and his fear that they will be too much for the clinician to bear. Having established this is the patient's perception there is simply more gentle probing aimed at helping him talk about what is troubling him.

The importance of containing the person's difficult feelings cannot be over-emphasised. If the person becomes physiologically aroused, the cognitive impact is that s/he will find it harder to think and participate fully. Moreover, this may lead her/him to cognitively interpret that arousal in ways that increase the likelihood of dangerous behaviours.

Therefore, as you probe deeper, you always need to be thinking of both how you are responding, remaining composed, and how you can help the person express difficult feelings without becoming psychologically and physiologically overwhelmed.

Keeping the interview moving
Although an assessment should have a drive towards seeking solutions and has much therapeutic value in itself, it is still using time to elicit information. Because of this, an important skill lies in knowing what information is likely to be important and how to keep the interview moving without the person feeling you are trivialising her/his experience, are disinterested or simply following your own agenda. Means of attempting to keep the interview moving in a positive sense, having already conveyed the purpose of the meeting and how much time you actually have to devote to it, are as follows.

- Find out what the patient wants and why.
- Align yourself with the patient's agenda, i.e. concern yourself with what is important to her/him and what s/he wants (without colluding or making promises you are not in a position to keep).

- Keep the process, and your language, simple.
- Avoid jargon and 'psychiatric-speak', e.g. 'Your levels of observation are…' or 'I am going to be your keyworker'.
- Having established clarity about your own boundaries, maintain them.

Most importantly, particular to this person and her/his presentation and more generally, know what you must try to clearly elicit and prioritise according to the circumstances and the time available.

Key clinical tip

There may be very distressing incidents or issues which the patient has difficulty discussing. If there is an issue which you think is too difficult for the person to address at any stage of the assessment, or which might take so much time it could 'derail' the assessment process, you can 'log it' and move the assessment on.

Using different types of question

Any interview requires different types of questions, differing techniques and different approaches appropriate to the stage of the interview, what is being discussed and the dynamic changes in the relationship between the interviewer and interviewee. This is certainly true of a risk assessment with someone experiencing mental distress, potentially suicidal and/or violent.

Preparing for, and during, an assessment, the assessor is continually thinking about how to ask questions, which questions to ask, and when. This process within the assessment will also be shaped by the use of any structured risk assessment tool. As stated above, however, perhaps the best approach is to have a clear understanding of the structure of a risk assessment, the information you need to elicit and then wrap that around the story the person provides. This makes the assessment more conversational, with questions flowing from previous answers.

It is also important to cultivate the ability to adapt, improvise and use different types of questions in response to something important mentioned by the person being assessed or if the person is finding the assessment more difficult than perhaps you'd expected.

Despite the views of some textbooks, there is not a 'perfect order' in which to use particular types of questions. Working out which question to use, and when, is as much a part of the assessment as anything.

Thus, open questions usually elicit more information and provide a better perspective of what it is like from the person's perspective, as they have the space to explore different themes in response to a non-specific question, e.g. 'How are you feeling?.'

Sometimes, however, asking closed questions can prove more helpful. For someone distressed, withdrawn, overwhelmed or pre-occupied it can be difficult to respond to a request to describe their broad feelings but much easier to formulate an answer to a simpler question, e.g. 'Have you been having trouble sleeping over the past two weeks?'.

Once the interview is flowing, it would be normal to move from open questions to 'funnelling in', to closed, specific questions, using a number of techniques to support this process. Below are types of questions and techniques you might use, with clinical examples.

Phrasing the question
What to ask, and when, can be crucial.

- Be specific when necessary – there will be times in the interview when it is necessary, especially when stating your concerns and understanding of the risk.
- Avoid ambiguity.
- Be brief in your questions.
- Use short silences, even if you feel uncomfortable doing so – allow the patient (and yourself) time to think and respond.

Open, non-specific questions
These are best used initially, e.g. 'How do you feel?', 'What has been happening?' or 'Tell me about yourself...'. Gradually, some focus can then be added, e.g. 'Tell me more about when you feel hopeless', or 'Are there times when you don't feel like that?'. However, also see section 3.4 above.

Closed questions
These elicit 'yes', 'no' or 'don't know' as an answer and can be used to provide an explicit focus and facilitate specific responses to areas of assessment where it is required. These are necessary when particular,

specific information is required. Examples are: 'Do you still feel like harming yourself?' or 'Did you want to die when you took the tablets?'. If the response is 'I don't know' or 'I'm not sure', further probing is obviously required.

Other interview techniques

Funnelling in
This is crucial in building on the information that has been gained in the interview from open and non-specific questions. There will be key points you want to focus on but this should be done gradually, using each question to bring you closer to the specifics of the main area of risk to the patient.

Clinical example 3: Funnelling in

Clinician: You said you were feeling desperate last night. Can you tell me more about that?

William: I'd had enough. Kelly had left. Everything had gone wrong.

Clinician: What had gone wrong?

William: Everything. There was my dad's death … I felt terrible. I just felt like I couldn't carry on anymore.

Clinician: What did you do then?

William: I got the tablets.

Clinician: You said how you were feeling. What were you thinking?

William: Thinking? I don't know … That it wasn't fair. That I should do something.

Clinician: Was there something specific you were thinking you should do?

William: [*Silence*]

Clinician: You said you were thinking things weren't fair and that you should do something. What did you think you should do?

William: I … I couldn't face life anymore.

Clinician: Were you thinking about killing yourself?

William:	Yes.
Clinician:	Had you thought about how you would do that?
William:	Um, yes.
Clinician:	What was your plan?
William:	To go to the station and throw myself under a train.
Clinician:	Was there a reason you thought about that particularly?
William:	How do you mean?
Clinician:	Well, I was wondering why you would think specifically of throwing yourself under a train? Had you thought about other ways in which to kill yourself but then decided against them?
William:	I took tablets before but that hadn't worked. That's why I started thinking about a train. I know there are fast trains that come through the station and ... and that would be it.
Clinician:	That sounds very definite. What stopped you following through on your plan?
William:	I'm not sure. I did go down there, once, then came home. I was thinking about the driver of the train, you know, what it would be like ... And I started thinking about my family having to see me ... I just reached the stage where I couldn't think anymore. The tablets were there and I just took them.
Clinician:	So, although you took them on the spur of the moment, you'd definitely been thinking about it and had something of a plan?
William:	Yes.

Seeking clarification

It is easy to think that we understand the person's perspective or that we understand the motivation for risk behaviours. The pattern of behaviour that led to it might appear obvious and fit within a clearly established pattern. For example, looking in from outside we may perceive the individual's pattern as their contact with mental health services diminishes; having been 'well' for a while, s/he questions the need for prescribed medication and takes it less regularly; an increase in stress leads to poor sleep and pronounced social anxiety; the person attempts to self-medicate using illicit drugs; psychotic symptoms worsen and risk behaviours occur.

However, what is important in an assessment is to go on a journey with the person and understand how they understand their situation, what they see as the problems and the precipitants. While this applies to the entire thrust of the interview, it is crucial in the detail of the discussion. Seeking clarification is, therefore, an ideal opportunity to see whether or not you have understood what has been said to date, display active listening and continue to build a rapport.

Clinical example 4: Seeking clarification

William: I'm fed up with you lot, always 'doing things' to me.

Clinician: Us lot? Do you mean myself and Jenny?

William: You know. You lot. You've been doing things to me for 15 years now.

Clinician: I'm still not sure who you mean when you say, 'You lot'. Could you help me out?

William: Nurses. Doctors. Filling me with injections, doing things to my head.

Clinician: So not specifically me and Jenny?

William: You're all the same.

Clinician: It sounds like you feel you've not been helped by nurses and psychiatrists in the past. Maybe we can talk about that and how we can try and find something that's helpful for you now, rather than things happening that you don't want or that aren't helpful.

When talking about risk, it is always important to be as specific as possible and, if there is any doubt, to seek clarification.

Clinical example 5: Seeking clarification

Clinician: You were saying just now that you thought the tablets you took would kill you.

William: Yes.

Clinician: And a few times you've said that you wanted to escape. As I understand it, you were referring to wanting to escape the situation you'd found yourself in. Is that right?

William: And the feelings. I just couldn't bear being in so much pain and not able to see any way out, you know?

Clinician: Well, I'm not quite sure I do. Do you mean that you wanted to die? Or was dying the only way out, the only way to escape, that you could see?

William: Yeah. There is no other way out. That's obvious.

Clinician: So it isn't actually that you want to die. You want to escape.

William: But ... well, maybe...

Clinician: Let me put it another way, if there were something that would get you out of the situation and help you feel 'better', that didn't mean you had to die, would you want that?

William: Yes. [*Pause*] But there's not, is there?

Clinician: That's something we can talk about.

Reflection

Occasionally, it may be useful to reflect on a comment made by the person, because you feel it is important and want to emphasise it, that you want to 'pause' the progress of the interview to get more information about the point that has arisen or make an empathic comment. Often, reflection is validating for the person.

Clinical example 6: Reflection

Simple reflection

William: There's just times when I've completely had enough.
Clinician: Had enough?
William: You know, like when Kelly left. I knew I couldn't cope and I thought about killing myself.

Reflecting and challenging

William: … and everything is going wrong and there's just no point because whatever I do … well …
Clinician: Everything goes wrong?
William: Yeah. Absolutely.
Clinician: Yet when we were talking earlier you spoke about your relationship with your mother and brother and how much that meant to you, how you'd helped them with so many things. I've got that right, haven't I?
William: Maybe. It doesn't feel like that now though.
Clinician: Yes, I got that impression.

Getting no response

If you don't get a response or the interview seems to be 'stuck' it is worth reflecting on what has happened.

- Was the question too threatening?
- Did the patient understand the question?
- Was it the 'right' question for that stage of the interview?
- Options are to:
    - rephrase the question;
    - gently 'nudge' the patient;
    - leave it and return to it later.

If the person doesn't respond, you should directly address this rather than ignore it.

Clinical example 7: No response from the patient

Leave it and return later

Clinician: You don't seem comfortable with this issue.
Michael: No, I'm not.
Clinician: Would you rather we come back to it later?
Michael: Yes.

Rephrasing

Clinician: How did it help your feelings of anger when you punched Daniel?
Michael: [*Silence*]
Clinician: When you look back on it now, how do you feel about what happened between you and Daniel?

Gently 'nudging'

Clinician: How did it help your feelings of anger when you punched Daniel?
Michael: [*Silence*]
Clinician: I get the sense this is a difficult subject for you, but I think it would be helpful for both you and me if we can try and understand what happened.

Confronting

Sometimes, a clinician has to be even more forthright. Often this involves making an observation. Wherever possible, you should convey the view of the clinical team but, at the same time 'own' the response with an 'I' message, so that it is clear to the person that talking to you has value and that s/he is clear about your views (see example 2 in Clinical example 8 below).

Clinical example 8: Confronting

Example 1

Clinician: You're telling me everything's okay and that I should let you leave the ward for a while, but, I have to be honest, William, looking at you now, it doesn't seem as if much has changed from when you came in yesterday. You look as if you're feeling very distressed and I get the impression you're still feeling very low.

Example 2

Clinician: I know you want to leave but I'm afraid I don't feel it would be safe to let you. The team have been very concerned about you and just now I'd like you to remain on the ward.

Bringing a solution-focused approach

Even in an assessment with an individual apparently in the midst of a terrible crisis, beset by problems, it is possible to explore solutions. This should not be confused with solution-focused therapy and the solution-focused assessment that is undertaken as part of this model. However, simple questions, once the degree of the problem(s) has been ascertained, allow the person to think about her/his earlier coping mechanism, problem-solving techniques and psychological strengths.

Clinical example 9: A solution-focused approach

Example 1

William: I don't think anyone can understand what this is like. I can't see how I can sort any of it out. It's such a mess.

Clinician: This is obviously really difficult for you. But has anything helped you in the past when you've felt like this?

Example 2

William: What am I going to do? I've failed at everything I've tried to do and I'm not surprised Kelly had enough and went. I'm useless.

Clinician: Given all that's happened, with your father dying, losing your job, Kelly and you splitting up, I think you've done remarkably well to cope as well as you have up until now. How did you do that?

It is important that you are able to communicate clearly that you are not minimising the person's perception of their difficulties. Also, it needs to be remembered that someone who is depressed and suicidal will find problem-solving extremely difficult, not just about practical matters but also when it comes to looking forward, to relationship issues and dealing with more abstract things, and will need to be guided through the process of how to do this.

Closing down difficult issues during the interview

There will be times when you do not want to explore an issue that comes up in an assessment. This might be for a number of reasons.

- You do not think you have the expertise to do so.
- You may decide it is going to take you too far from the core issues of risk you need to assess within a given time.
- You may be concerned that exploring it now, within the context of the assessment, will lead to the person becoming too aroused and distressed, possibly jeopardising the opportunity to complete the assessment.

There are a number of ways in which you can 'close down' the issue while still communicating some important points, including:

- that you have 'heard' something important the person wants to tell you;
- that you do not think this is the right time to discuss it – and why;
- what you are going to do about this.

Clinical example 10: Closing down

Example 1: Discussing the issue and then drawing it to a close

Clinician: So, by the sounds of it, you're not someone who has lots of friends and you haven't 'carried' them on through school and different jobs, and stayed in touch.

William: No, not really. I've got mates but I'm not really close to them.

Clinician: But people like your friend, Vicky, and your brother, have always been important to you and you've stayed very close with them?

William: Yeah, that's right.

Clinician: Thanks. Now we've talked about your friends, I'd like to ask you about your sexual relationships if that's okay.

William: Yes. All right.

Clinician: When did you have your first sexual relationship?

William: What, you mean like a proper partner?

Clinician: It may have been a long-term partner, but I was wondering about how old you were when you first had a sexual relationship.

William: Oh. Not until I was 21. I know it's quite old, isn't it?

[*Later in the interview*]

Clinician: Thank you for being so frank with me. It's been helpful. Moving on though, this is a question you may not feel comfortable to answer, but I have to ask. I was wondering if you have ever felt abused in any way, possibly physically, psychologically or sexually?

William: [*Long pause*] I told you about my mother's boyfriend, after she and my dad split up? That was when … when things started to happen, when he came into the house and I was on my own.

[*Later in the interview*]

Clinician: That was obviously a very upsetting time and I get the impression it was difficult for you to talk about it. I don't want to ignore it but, because we have to finish fairly soon, I'd like to move on to talk about what happened last night, when you took the tablets. If you want to talk more about these issues, we can agree a time and talk about it later rather than try to carry on now and not be able to give it the time it needs. Would that be okay with you?

William: Yeah. That's … um, well, it's still really upsetting but I'd feel okay talking about it another time.

Example 2: An issue arises and the clinician doesn't feel fully competent to address it

William: That was when … when things started to happen, when my mum's boyfriend came into the house and I was on my own.

Clinician: I understand it might be important for you to talk about this but, to be honest, it's not an area in which I have a lot of experience. I'm going to ask one of my colleagues if they can talk more with you about this later. It's not that I don't want to help, but I think you'd benefit more from talking with someone who has more experience.

Example 3: An issue arises which might deter from the risk assessment

William: It's like when I start thinking about stuff … about things that happened when my mum's boyfriend came into the house… when she wasn't there…

Clinician: This is obviously distressing for you. I also get the sense that it's important but I think it might be better to focus on what was happening when you decided to take the tablets and then return to it after, if you feel okay about that?

Digression

As noted above, while having an internalised assessment structure, knowledge of what information you are seeking and what types of questions and interview techniques to use at different stages of the assessment, it is a high-level skill to be able to facilitate the person digressing while being able to bring it back to the core issues with the assessment. In Clinical example 11, using Michael's case study (below), we see the clinician exploring further elements of his psychotic thinking before returning to the central theme of exploring a recent assault on another patient.

Clinical example 11: Digression

Clinician: So it was when you thought Daniel did something to you that you decided you would hit him?

Michael: I didn't just think it. You're like all the others. You reckon this is all in my head.

Clinician: I'm sorry. I didn't mean to convey that impression. Could you tell me what happened?

Michael: He's been at it for ages and you all let him. You don't care.

Clinician: I'm not sure what you mean. Could you explain?

Michael: No. Why should I?

Clinician: [*Silence*]

Michael: He's been trying to infect me, hasn't he? Like you lot.

Clinician: Us lot?

Michael: You know. Some of the nurses do it as well.

Clinician: Try to infect you?

Michael: Yeah.

Clinician: How does that work?

Michael: Putting their thoughts into me. Wanting me to do things. Take my powers away.

Clinician: What's the reason Daniel and these nurses do that?

Michael: Because they're scared of me, of course.

Clinician: What are they scared of? Something you could do?

Michael: Just my powers. I can do anything if I want. They think I'd hurt them. But I wouldn't. Not unless they start attacking me like Daniel did.

Clinician: Do you know how they do this? The infecting, I mean.

Michael: No, not really. It's like they do it with their thoughts.

Clinician: So how do you know when it's happening?

Michael: 'Cause I can feel it. My heart starts going a bit faster. Things start happening in my gut. I feel like something's been put in my legs, like I can't stand still but my feet go funny, spongy like.

Clinician: Was that happening just before you hit Daniel?

Michael: Yeah.

Clinician: And was that why you hit him, or was it because of the cigarettes?

Michael: I'm not worried about the cigarettes. I could've got those back. It did annoy me a bit and I might have done him because of that. But it was this infecting thing. I'm not having it, am I?

Summarising

During the course of a risk assessment it is often useful to pause to reflect on what information has emerged and how you have understood it. Remembering that the person's cognitive functioning is likely to be impaired by anxiety and psychological arousal, it provides an opportunity to remind her/him of what has been said up until that point. It also allows you to:

- state the key points as you've understood them from the discussion so far;
- check if everything is clear between yourself and the patient;
- see if you have missed anything;
- check if the person wants to add anything;
- discuss what comes next, given the point reached at this stage of the interview.

Clinical example 12: Summarising

Clinician: It might be useful if we pause for a moment to summarise where we have got to. As I understand it, from what you've said, this has been a very difficult few months, with pressures at work, your father's death and you not sleeping well. You felt Kelly leaving was the last straw and that was when you started to think about killing yourself. Is that right?

William: Kind of. Things hadn't been right between me and Kelly for a while. And I think I was maybe drinking a bit too much sometimes. Not much. But sometimes. I know Kelly didn't like it.

Clinician: Okay. I think I missed that. Thanks. It's useful and maybe we'll come back to that a bit later? Just now I wondered if we could talk a bit more about the thoughts you were having about killing yourself?

William: Do we have to?

Clinician: I think it would be helpful if we could.

Genuineness

If you can utilise the skills outlined above and combine them with something of your own personality, this can be very useful in helping develop a rapport and moving the risk assessment process forward.

Stuart (2005: 35) has described genuineness in the nurse-patient relationship as, '[t]he nurse is an open, honest and sincere person who is actively involved in the relationship'. This is achieved by the nurse thinking and feeling the same thing, not suppressing feelings and, most importantly, saying the same thing(s) as s/he is thinking and feeling.

To this, perhaps, can be added something else. In focusing on the person being assessed and what s/he is saying, being mindful of that person, you are more likely to respond to her/him rather than thinking about what you 'should' say in the circumstances. Undoubtedly, this is partly about confidence, which in turn comes from having experience and knowing something about how you cope under pressure. It is also about feeling confident enough to bring something of your own personality into the process, to know when and how much it is appropriate to self-disclose (see 'Self-disclosure' section below), using your own 'voice' while remembering that you are also trying to tap into the language of the person you're assessing.

Concreteness
This is an essential communications tool used in developing and maintaining therapeutic relationships. In the context of risk assessment it involves being specific, particularly when discussing the patient's feelings, experiences and behaviours. It 'avoids vagueness and ambiguity and is the opposite of generalising, labelling, and making assumptions about the patient's experience', all essential in formulating a good risk assessment (Stuart 2005: 37).

Respect
Respect encompasses politeness, aspects of empathy and genuineness. Although it may seem a very simple thing, and something that is trotted out in many nursing texts, to be respectful of someone who behaves in a very challenging manner or who has done things that go against your own ethical or moral codes is never easy. It involves accepting the person for who s/he is, being able to listen to, and accept, their story neutrally, with curiosity and without exhibiting judgement or criticism. Behaviours, feeling and attitudes are accepted as 'natural' or 'normal' given the circumstances the person finds her/himself in.

Our own attitudes and experience – both clinical and personal – will affect how we feel towards individual patients, as well as what has been happening on the day we meet them. As mentioned earlier in this text, conducting a complex risk assessment does not happen in a vacuum. If you have already been involved in several difficult assessments or have particular concerns about an earlier patient, or even things that have happened outside work, these will all impact upon your capacity to think and feel your way through the process you are engaged in with this individual.

The importance of respect in assessing and managing risk is that it both acknowledges the potential for change as and when circumstances are different, and makes it easier for the person to tell her/his story, particularly those parts of it that have been very distressing and/or disturbing.

A clinician displaying personal attributes such as respect and politeness may also make it easier for the person to accept things that might provoke a more challenging reaction otherwise.

Self-disclosure

This can be another brick in helping you build a relationship with the person you are assessing. Knowing what and how much to disclose is never easy but should reflect a genuine, respectful and empathic relationship with the person and have a therapeutic purpose, e.g. to model something, be educative, validate feelings or develop the therapeutic alliance you are attempting to foster.

Clinical example 13: Self-disclosure

Clinician: So things between Kelly and yourself were difficult for a while?

William: Yes. [*Pause*] Are you married?

Clinician: Yes, I've been married for several years.

William: You don't wear a ring.

Clinician: I broke my finger a few years ago and the joint swells, so I can't put it on anymore. Why do you ask?

William: I don't know. You look as if you might be.

Clinician: Are you wondering if I can understand your situation?

William: I doubt you've got a relationship like I had with Kelly.

Clinician: If you tell me about your relationship with Kelly then perhaps I can understand?

In this example the clinician doesn't avoid the question but uses it as an opportunity to explore William's feelings, not only about his relationship with his wife but also how much he feels understood in the assessment.

Things to avoid

Avoid leading questions

Leading questions and assumptions can cause all sorts of problems. If the information has not yet been established, e.g. whether or not the person actually intended to kill himself, don't ask, 'Why did you want to kill yourself?' Instead, ask 'Did you want to kill yourself?'.

Avoid multiple questions

For example, 'Do you have trouble getting off to sleep or wake up early? What do you think about when you can't sleep?'. This is actually three separate questions:

- Do you have trouble getting off to sleep?
- Do you wake up early?
- What do you think about when you can't sleep?

Not validating the person's experience

This is quite difficult, particularly if the person you are assessing is psychotic, and requires some thought, accepting the person's story as s/he explains it.

Clinical example 14: Not validating the person's experience

Clinician: Tell me more about these ideas you get about Daniel and others infecting you.

Michael: You're like all the others. You don't believe me. They're not ideas. It's real. There's no point talking to you. I'm going.

Such a situation as that in Clinical example 14 (above) can potentially be avoided by adopting a different way of exploring the issue.

Clinical example 15: Validating the person's experience

Clinician: Tell me more about what happened between you and Daniel.

Michael: What, the infecting thing?

Clinician: Yes.

Michael: He does it to wind me up and because he's scared of me.

Clinician: And do you get wound up?

Michael: Of course. Anyone would.

Clinician: What happens to you when you're wound up?

Michael: I have to do things.

Clinician: What sort of things?

Michael: I don't know … I have to get rid of the feeling. What it's like. Being wound up.

Clinician: What does it feel like?

Michael: It's horrible. Like everything inside me is rigid and there's loads of energy buzzing through me but my head's full of stuff and I can't think. I feel all sweaty and I just want them to stop it.

Clinician: It does sound horrible, a bit like things feel out of control.

Michael: Exactly.

In this example, the clinician hasn't colluded with Michael's belief that other patients can 'infect' him and that is the source of his psychological and physiological state of arousal. But by asking Michael more about what he believes to be happening and then validating Michael's feelings related to his experience, he is able to elicit crucial information that progresses his risk assessment, particularly in relation to Michael feeling threatened and that things are out of his control.

Closing, or finishing, the assessment interview

This is a vital part of the interview when you will seek to summarise and consolidate all that you have discussed in your time with the patient. It should incorporate a discussion about the key issues that have arisen, including risks, an attempt to understand the context of these risks (very similar to a clinical formulation but in the individual's own language) and move on to a plan for future contact and risk management (see Table 3.3).

Clinical example 16: Closing the session

Clinician: Thanks, William, for discussing so much with me, particularly as there were some things it was clearly very hard to talk about.

William: Yes, well … it's been helpful, I guess.

Clinician: I just wanted to go over the key things as I understood them. Is that OK?

William: Yeah.

Clinician: From what you were saying, it's been a very difficult few months, since your father's death…

William: I'd been struggling before that, when he was ill … you know, like I said…

Clinician: Yes, I was going to come to that. But it seems as if you felt much worse after his death, less able to cope with the sort of things you'd been managing to do previously. Is that right?

William: Yeah, and then Kelly…

Clinician: And after Kelly left you began having more thoughts about suicide, and then took the tablets with the intention of killing yourself?

William: [Looks down at the floor and nods]

Clinician: But this had been building for a long time…

William: My whole life, it seems now.

Clinician: Yes, you were saying it had brought up a lot of stuff from when you were very young, as well as your first marriage and things you've struggled with for a long time.

William: [Nods again]

Clinician: So we've agreed that, because you're still having very strong thoughts about killing yourself and aren't sure that you'll be able to resist them, particularly if you're back at the flat on your own and even with people coming in to see you, you'll come into hospital for a short period of time while we look at how we can help you look at other options. We'll start that anti-depressant we discussed but also think about how to help you look again at some of the problems you've identified.

William: I can't really think much more. I feel exhausted.

Clinician: I know. While we arrange to take you into hospital I'm going to get you a drink and sandwich if you'd like one. I'll also give you a copy of that plan, or agreement, we talked about so you can have a look at it when you're ready. It lists the things we'll do to try to help, as I explained, as well as the things you thought you could do. I'll also get the leaflets about the ward and medication. I know it's a lot, and I don't expect you to take it all in just now. It will be there so you can look at them in your own time when you've had a chance to rest a bit.

Table 3.3 Closing the session – key points

Summarise the content of the interview.
Summarise what has been agreed.
Particularly focus on any risk management plan.
Make clear who will do what, e.g. patient and clinician to 'manage' risks.
Ensure the person has nothing else to ask or clarify.
Provide a reminder of what will happen with information, e.g. documentation.
Agree what will happen next, e.g. next appointment or meeting.

Risk assessment in the context of a full mental health assessment

So far, we have explored interviewing someone either already well known to you or your service where the key requirement is a risk assessment in the context of the person's current circumstances. The structure of this interview is relatively straightforward: what happened, what was the person thinking/feeling, what did the person want to happen etc. However, there are times when a risk assessment, or re-assessment, is required as part of a full mental health assessment. An example would be when meeting someone not previously known to you or the service.

It could also include someone who has not been assessed for a period during which there could have been significant changes, perhaps due to the time since they were last assessed or simply something about how the person now sees their experience.

There are numerous ways in which to construct a mental health assessment and, in part, these might be defined by the use of specific assessment tools, e.g. KGV-M Assessment Tool, the Carers and Users Expectation of Services (CUES), Beck's Depression Inventory, Liverpool University Neuroleptic Side Effects Rating Scale (LUNSERS), while there are also tools that can be used to assist the risk assessment process, including the Galatean Risk Screening Tool (GRIST), Historical Clinical Risk-20 (HCR-20), Short Term Assessment of Risk and Treatability (START), Sexual Violence Risk-20 (SVR-20) and Violence Risk Appraisal Guide (VRAG) (Department of Health 2007).

However, while the risk assessment essentially remains the same, the placing of it within the interview process is crucial and this guide suggests a structure that aims to build a full picture of the individual and all aspects of her/his history before addressing risk as a specific issue, thus beginning with 'the history of the presenting complaint' and ending with risk.

There are obviously huge numbers of texts that offer advice and the evidence base for undertaking a mental health assessment and mental state examination. This *Pocket Guide* is not going to replicate these but will focus on different components of the assessment as they *potentially* relate to risk.

Appearance and behaviour

As stressed throughout the *Pocket Guide*, what you see is very important, particularly in terms of congruence, and the first part of a mental state examination is actually to note how the person appears and behaves during the interview. In particular, thinking of motivation and a willingness to collaborate with the process of risk management:

- Does the person volunteer information, or is s/he elusive or finds it difficult to articulate her/his experience?
- Is there anything to indicate the person's level of self-care, e.g. have they washed, are their clothes clean?
- How is s/he dressed?
- What is the person's facial expression?
- Has s/he any distinctive marks, scars, tattoos etc.?
- What is the person's emotional and cognitive state *during* the interview? Does it vary? Is there anything particular that is distressing? Does the person appear distracted, preoccupied etc.?
- Is s/he restless?
- Do her/his reactions and responses seem appropriate, in your opinion, to the situation (it is important to stress that this area of assessment is highly subjective)?

History of presenting complaint

This involves identifying the background to issues leading to presentation. The approach is partly determined by the circumstances that led to the presentation, particularly its urgency. However, to establish clarity, it's important to set some parameters, e.g. 'Tell me what brought you here now'.

The key words 'here' and 'now' get more information about what brought the patient to you now.

Clinical example 17: Focusing on the immediate reasons the person is being assessed

Clinician: Tell me what brought you here now.

William: Well, I'm feeling pretty depressed.

Clinician: I'm sorry to hear that. How long have you been depressed?

William: I don't know. Years. Most of my life really.

Clinician: OK. What was different that you came here today?

William: I haven't been able to sleep. I'm feeling a lot more anxious … It feels like it's getting worse.

Clinician: What might have changed recently that you've been feeling like that?

Key clinical tip

Focusing on the 'here' and 'now' at the start of the risk assessment provides focus and allows you to gain an understanding of the immediate problem(s).

Full biographical history

It is easy to assume we 'know' a person, her/his experience and can understand what is happening with them, especially when there is a lot of documentation about that person, either in the form of reports or previous assessments. However, nothing can be as useful as hearing from the person about how they understand and relate their experience.

For example, contrast these two comments from patients diagnosed with schizophrenia, both based on actual clinical sessions.

Clinical example 18: Exploring the person's sense of himself

Example 1

Clinician: Hi, Michael, thanks for seeing me [*explains assessment process*]. OK, so maybe you could begin by telling me about yourself.

Michael: Well, there's nothing much to say [*pause*]. I don't know, I'm Michael and I'm schizophrenic.

Clinician: OK. Where were you born?

Michael: London.

Clinician: Is that where your family were from?

Michael: No.

Clinician: Are you OK talking about these things with me, Michael?

Michael: Yeah. But I don't see the point. It's not going to change what happened or who I am.

Example 2

Clinician: Hi, Simon, thanks for seeing me [*explains assessment process*]. OK, so maybe you could begin by telling me about yourself.

Simon: I'm not sure what I should say.

Clinician: Why not start with your parents and your family, where they were from, what they did…

Simon: Oh. Well, I was born in London but my mum is Irish and she met my dad in Liverpool. That's where he's from. They came down to London after they married because of my dad's job. And my sister, Jo, had just been born.

Clinician: What did your dad do?

Simon: He worked as a teacher but he got a better job, I think, or more money or something. I know my mum used to say she wished they'd stayed in Liverpool. She had family up there but didn't know anyone here. I think she found it hard to fit in, make friends and things and my dad was busy because of his job.

From the outset, Michael states that his personal identity is tied up with his diagnosed 'illness' and intimates that nothing is going to change. This contrasts with Simon, who has a sense of his family, relationships and feelings within the family. Although they are very different starting points, and suggest very different personal narratives, it is from here that you can begin to explore:

- Who is this person?
- How does s/he see her/himself?
- How do these events fit into her/his life?
- The details of her/his family, education, employment, social, economic, relationship and sexual history.
- Take a full medical and psychiatric history.
- Gather details about all drug and alcohol use.
- Get details of any forensic history – not just asking if the patient has been in trouble with the police or has convictions, but:
    - Has s/he done anything that might have resulted in police action?
    - Has s/he been involved in acts of violence in the past?
    - Has s/he used weapons?
    - Does s/he carry weapons?

There are obviously difficult areas to negotiate here but, if the flow of the questions relates to the person's story and has progressed reasonably well, it is best to address them in a very straightforward manner (see clinical examples 19 and 20).

One of the most daunting areas for less experienced clinicians, however, is the issue of a full psychosexual history. It can feel intrusive and not as important as other 'things'. In particular, there may be an anxiety about sexual abuse being disclosed or, if it has in previous assessments, being spoken about. There is, nonetheless, crucial information in this area of a person's life and, given its relationship to risks such as self-harm, abuse is one of those. It may be, as well, that the person being assessed may have been abusive in relationships but, even if abuse is absent, sex and sexual relationships are an important part of most people's lives and warrant exploration.

As is discussed later, an assessment is not a therapy session and you probably won't have the time to explore abuse in any depth. Nor is it appropriate or helpful to bring it out into the open and then 'leave it', so it does take some skill to ask about it and then leave the person feeling heard while being able to gently close it down with an indication of what you will do with the information divulged (see clinical example 10).

As with any potentially difficult areas of the assessment, building towards it helps the person, while the offer of 'opting out' of answering should remain. Thus, in exploring relationships, you start by asking about friendships from the local area, school, university, work etc. then ask about sexual relationships. It gives the person being assessed some continuity and a logical progression. It also makes it easier to then move on to asking if the person feels s/he has ever been abused in any way, including physically, psychologically or sexually.

In conclusion, you cannot expect someone to necessarily divulge their most intimate secrets when first meeting you. However, genuine curiosity within a framework that is compassionate and concerned can be very effective. A full biographical history is important in risk assessments in that it's only through the individual's life and her/his account of it that you can fully understand the idiosyncrasies and important events that have shaped them, their psyche and their attitudes to issues of risk.

Clinical example 19: Addressing risk to others

Clinician: Thanks for that. I want to move on, if that's OK?
Michael: Yeah.
Clinician: You mentioned that you got in some trouble when you were at school. Did that involve the police?
Michael: What, like being arrested?
Clinician: Yes.
Michael: No.
Clinician: Was that the sort of thing – or has there been anything else – that might have got you in trouble with the police if it had come to their attention?
Michael: [*Pause*] I'm not sure what you mean.
Clinician: Maybe getting into fights or doing anything illegal. That kind of thing.
Michael: [*Pause*] I did a bit of shoplifting when I was a kid.
Clinician: What sort of things?
Michael: Just stuff. Nothing much.
Clinician: Was it for you or stuff you could sell?
Michael: Bit of both.

Clinician: How did you get into that?

Michael: An older kid used to do it and he showed me the ropes.

Clinician: Did you always do it together?

Michael: No. He used to keep everything for himself so I went off on my own.

Clinician: You were saying earlier that you've used a lot of cannabis and cocaine in the past but hadn't been able to find work. Did you ever have to steal things so you could buy drugs?

Michael: A bit. Everyone does that.

Clinician: Did you ever sell drugs so you could buy your own?

Michael: Maybe. I can't remember. Anyway, I cut right down. I knew it was getting out of hand.

Clinician: Were there any other things?

Michael: Ah, I had one or two arguments. But nothing serious.

Clinician: Did they ever become physical?

Michael: A couple of times. Only to defend myself. If I was being threatened, you know?

Clinician: What happened?

Michael: This guy was going to do things to me.

Clinician: How did you know that? Was it something he said?

Michael: He didn't have to.

Clinician: But you knew?

Michael: Oh yeah. The way he was looking, the way he was standing.

Clinician: That told you?

Michael: Yeah. You'd know, wouldn't you? If someone was going to do something to you?

Clinician: I'm not sure. What sort of things did you think he was going to do?

Michael: Mess up my head. Infect me.

Clinician: And how would he be able to do that?

Michael: Put stuff in me. I don't know.

Clinician: What did you do?

Michael: Hit him.

Clinician: Did you punch him or use a weapon?

Michael: I punched him a couple of times … He'd really been getting at me, you know? So I s'pose I gave him a bit of a kicking when he went down. Then I ran off before anyone could grab me.

Clinician: Is that what led to you coming into hospital?

Michael: Not really. I was stitched up by my CPN. He told the psychiatrist and social worker stuff about me that wasn't true.

Clinician: OK, so there have been a few incidents when you've felt you needed to defend yourself and that led to you hitting people. [*Pause*] Have you ever used a weapon?

Michael: Only to defend myself.

Clinician: What did you use?

Michael: I used a strap wrapped around my fist. It makes it more painful when you hit them and you don't hurt your hand as much. I hit someone with a bottle once but it didn't break. In fact I hit him twice. And he had a right hard head. I got a good kicking for that.

Clinician: When was that?

Michael: About two years ago. I haven't done anything like that since.

Clinician: Until the incident in the pub?

Michael: Yeah.

Clinician: What happened on that occasion?

Michael: Same thing. He was going to start doing things. He knew my mum and where I grew up and everything about me. He was jealous of what I've done and what I've got. His girlfriend was staring at me, like she could see what I was thinking, you know, about fancying her and what I was thinking of doing to her. So I hit her first.

Clinician: And was it the same when you hit the man in the pub with a bottle?

Michael: [*Laughs*] No, that was over a girl. She was nice though.

Clinician: Were you seeing her?

Michael: No, I fancied her but she was going out with him and I had a go at him 'cause he didn't like me talking to her.

Clinician: Have you ever felt you needed to carry a weapon?

Michael: [*Pause*] Sometimes.

Clinician: What was happening that you needed to do that?

Michael: In case someone was after me.

Clinician: Was that a concern about anyone in particular?

Michael:	No. It could have been anyone. That's why I needed to protect myself.
Clinician:	So what did you carry with you?
Michael:	It was only one of those jack-knife things. You know, one you can open up. I never had to use it.
Clinician:	Do you think you would have used it?
Michael:	Only if I had to. You know, like if anyone is trying to do stuff to me, like mess up my head. I wouldn't have used it against someone like that clown in the pub.
Clinician:	Why did you stop carrying it with you?
Michael:	I nearly got stopped by the police a couple of times so I threw it in the river. I didn't want to get nicked.
Clinician:	How did you manage to feel safe without it?
Michael:	I didn't really. I was always on edge, you know? I had to be really careful about where I went and who was about.
Clinician:	Is that when you started using cannabis a bit more.
Michael:	Yeah. It helped. Took the edge off things. Chilled me.

In this lengthy example, the clinician simply follows the story without commenting on the behaviours or indicating any personal views about it, which enables him to gather more information. From this, the clinician now has a clear understanding of the motivating factors for Michael's violence and a number of risks are elicited:

1. Michael has a history of violent assaults on strangers in response to psychotic phenomena but will also get into arguments and use violence when not psychotic.
2. He has routinely carried a weapon to protect himself and would have used it.
3. He has been involved in theft and the buying and selling of drugs.
4. He minimises his violence and other dangerous behaviours and doesn't readily volunteer information.
5. He displays no remorse for his violence.
6. He derives at least a degree of gratification or pleasure from his violence.

All of these factors, and the information gleaned in Clinical example 20, can now feature in the assessment of risk and its management.

Clinical example 20: Exploring attitudes to violence

Clinician: Thinking about the people you hit…

Michael: [*Interrupts*] It wasn't like I did it for nothing. It wasn't down to me. Besides, it's not a big deal. I hope you're not going to use this against me.

Clinician: Well, I need to share it with the team. But I did explain that at the beginning. I was wondering how you felt after you'd hit those people.

Michael: All right. How am I supposed to feel? They deserved it. I told you that. I was only defending myself.

Clinician: Did you enjoy it in any way?

Michael: [*Pause*] A bit, I suppose, now you ask. I never really thought that much about it. Not always.

Clinician: Do you know if any of them were badly hurt?

Michael: No. Well, I don't know, apart from the bloke I hit with the bottle. Even though the bottle didn't break, his head was still cut up. But his mates did me over for that, didn't they?

Key clinical tip

As well as helping establish a rapport before moving onto potentially more difficult topics, starting at 'the beginning' of someone's story, i.e. her/his family and very early background, establishes a chronological pattern to the interview, making it easier for the person to think about what is coming and feeling less 'surprised' by particular questions.

Mental state examination

This is a complex and detailed area of the assessment and there is not space to explore every aspect of it. Reference to further reading is detailed below while the broad content of a mental state examination is summarised in Table 3.4.

Table 3.4 Risk and the Mental State Examination (MSE)

Component of the MSE	What is being explored
Speech and language	• Fluency of speech (rate, volume, tone) • Pressure of speech • Content • Form
Thought: form	• Degree of connectedness • Continuity of thought • Formal thought disorder, e.g. loosening of association, knight's move thinking, word salad, thought block, perseveration and neologisms • Accelerated tempo of thought • Flight of ideas • Slowed tempo of thought • Psychic retardation • Goal-directedness • Linearity of thought
Thought: content	• Preoccupations • Ruminations • Obsessions • Topics • Phobias • Abnormal thoughts • Delusions or overvalued ideas • Thought interference, reference or persecution • Control or passivity • Thoughts of self-harm, suicide or homicide

Table 3.4 continued

Mood (the person's emotional state over a longer period of time) and **affect** (the emotional state of the person at a given moment in time)	**Objectively**, does the person appear: • elated • flat/blunted • incongruous • depressed or anxious • intense Is her/his mood reactive, for example does s/he smile when talking of something s/he enjoys? **Subjectively**, how does the person describe her/his mood? • Does this match your impression?
Perceptions	• Hallucinations, other perceptual disturbance
Cognitions	• Attention and concentration • Orientation to time, place and person • Level of comprehension • Short-term memory
Insight	• How does the person understand her/his experience? • Does s/he share the same views as others about her/his behaviour and its causes? • Does the person see her/his situation as unusual and due to changes in her/his mental state? Does s/he have some awareness that s/he may be different but have an alternative explanation for this?

Exploring the issues in Table 3.4 in detail is not always possible for various reasons. Perhaps it is a matter of time, perhaps the clinician given the responsibility for undertaking the risk assessment will not have been trained in taking a mental state examination (MSE) or have the experience. This does not preclude undertaking a risk assessment. Moreover, a full MSE may clearly be unnecessary.

However, if a formal MSE is not going to be part of the assessment process, you should nonetheless develop an understanding of how the person's mental state is impacting on potential issues of risk. For example:

- Is the person depressed?
- Is the person psychotic?
- Is their psychotic experience influencing their behaviour in a potentially dangerous way (see clinical example 19)?

It should be easier to then examine risk and understand how any feelings and ideas the person has about risk and risk behaviours fit into this person's life and current mental, psychological and emotional state.

Equally, if the person denies any ideas or plans about risk behaviours, there is more likely to be some evidence in the history for you to cite any concerns you have. For example, if the person has symptoms of clinical depression, describing difficulty in solving interpersonal problems, feeling trapped and seeing no hope for the future, yet then denies having even thought about suicide, the evidence base about depression and suicidal ideation would lead you to want to explore this more assertively.

Finally, having completed the assessment, you can then make a formulation and begin negotiating a plan (Harrison 2006).

Self-rating

Asking the person to rate how they feel, whether this be about their mood or another element of their clinical presentation, can be useful in getting an immediate sense of its severity. For example, considering thoughts about harming someone else can open up more detail about the risk, as well as allowing an insight into the decision-making process behind it.

Clinical example 21: Using a rating scale

Clinician: You were telling me that you had been thinking about hitting Daniel earlier.

Michael: Yeah.

Clinician: But you didn't feel like you had to do anything to him at that time?

Michael: No.

Clinician: What changed?

Michael: He started really staring at me. Like, right inside me. Like he wanted to eat my soul. Then he changed his mind and started all that infecting stuff and we had the argument ... it's hard to explain ... it was like I couldn't get the idea out of my head...

Clinician: I wonder if we can use a scale to help us work out the difference. Can you tell me how strong the thoughts were, on a scale of 1–10, with 1 being not strong at all and 10 meaning they couldn't have been any stronger? So, before the argument, how strong were they?

Michael: Well, I really didn't want to hit him. And I wasn't thinking about it that much, even though I'd made that threat. That was just my temper. So maybe 4 or 5.

Clinician: And what about after you noticed him staring at you?

Michael: That was different. Like I said, I couldn't stop thinking about it, even though I knew I shouldn't and ... well, I still didn't really want to...

Clinician: What number would you put to it?

Michael: 8. Maybe 9.

Clinician: That's a big jump. And that was why you went on to hit Daniel?

Michael: Yeah. Of course.

Clinician: At what number do you think the thoughts become so strong, that you're not going to be able to stop yourself from acting on them?

Michael: Um, I'm not sure. Maybe 7.

Clinician: So it sounds as if you carried on resisting for quite a while?

Michael: Yeah.

Clinician: Why was that?

Michael: I knew I'd get into trouble.

Clinician: Michael, this has really been useful in helping me understand what happens. I've just got a couple more questions.

Michael: Go on then.

Clinician: So once you get to 7, you're not going to be able to stop yourself?

Michael: No. I'm too wound up by then.

Clinician: And what number are you at most of the time?

Michael: [*Pause*] I don't know. That's a good question. Probably about 5.

Clinician: It doesn't take a lot to move you up to that point of no return then? You haven't a lot of space…

Michael: No. It's like I'm full up most of the time. That's the only way I can explain it.

Clinician: Maybe that's what we can work at – helping you feel less 'full'.

External factors

Considering the risks that might affect the person needs to encompass the world in which they find themselves, rather than an idealised situation or one that would be suited to their needs. Some of these factors may be quite idiosyncratic to the individual so it's impossible to provide an exhaustive list. However, these should figure in the clinician's thinking:

Environment and locality

What potential risks are in the wider environment? What, specifically, needs to be addressed, given that any environment will be host to a range of potential difficulties? For example, if substance misuse is a factor and there are drug dealers in the immediate neighbourhood, you need to consider how vulnerable the person is.

Equally, if prescribed medication is a crucial factor in the person remaining safe but they can't access a pharmacy without difficulty, that has to be factored into risk management.

Physical layout

If the person is being admitted to a ward, how suited is that to the level of security required for that person, particularly if s/he may try to abscond? For someone at risk of suicide, are there obvious ligature points or areas of the ward where the person would be alone for long periods and risks potentially increased?

Potential weapons

Almost any environment has a lot of potential weapons. Crucial questions are about what the person has used before, has talked about, and their intent. Avoiding interviews where the person has immediate access to more obvious – and potentially lethal – weapons such as knives or very sharp implements is discussed in 'The safety of the clinician and patient' section in Part 2 (page 51).

However, it is worth remembering that immediate access to a familiar, everyday object can be potentially lethal: picking up a frying pan in the midst of an argument and hitting someone across the head can occur in second, almost without thought.

Carers, friends and neighbours

(See also 'Working with families/carers and issues of confidentiality' in Part 2, page 56.)

Listening to the views of carers, relatives and friends is crucial. In countless suicide and homicide inquiry reports there are accounts of people having warned clinicians of their concerns about the patient but these concerns not being given sufficient weight (Appleby et al. 2006). Carers can also be an invaluable support and an integral part of a risk management plan. However, several factors need to be considered, including:

- Carers should not be over-burdened and given responsibilities for which they are either not ready or not able to carry out.
- The patient may not wish to receive their support at this time.
- The carer may be at risk.

Supporting the patient and carers can often be a difficult balancing act but it is important that this is part of the assessment and assumptions are not made.

Systems, service structures and procedures

As outlined in 'Key issues to determine from a risk assessment' in Part 1 (page 10) how our services are configured, access and availability will all be risk factors in themselves. Issues to consider include:

- If there is only a telephone triage system or helpline immediately available to the person, how will the assessor overcome the problems of not being able to see the person being assessed and compensate for the opportunity to assess body language, facial expression, congruity etc.?
- If the crisis team will have to risk assess a known patient 'outside hours' or when that person is in crisis, what access do they have to the latest information about the person?
- How will they know they are acting consistently with previous risk management plans?
- If there is pressure on beds, how do clinicians arrive at rational decisions based on the assessment of the individual?

Communication and coordination

How issues around the assessment are communicated and coordinated is central to the risk management plan. A 'plan', no matter how good, cannot be considered to exist if it is not communicated to, and understood by, the appropriate people. If there are flaws or problems in these crucial areas this will effectively nullify the impact of the assessment and increase risk. As such, the clinician needs to know how effective communications systems are and factor these into the plan. For example:

- If clinicians responsible for managing the risk won't have access to electronic records until the following day, how will information be passed on? By telephone? Fax? Is a physical meeting possible?
- If vital information has to be transmitted from one shift to another for several days, how will this be done?

 - Do nurses have time to read the electronic records of all patients?
 - Do you have a system for identifying the people about whom there is most concern?
 - Is this information displayed anywhere or is there a way of prioritising discussion to focus on them?
 - In an inpatient ward do you print off copies of safety care plans to ensure everyone can – and will – read them?
• If clinicians from a different team or service are to play an important role in the person's risk management, how will they know their specific responsibilities, what to do and what is in place in case things begin to go wrong?

If there are problems or, more specifically, gaps in any of these areas, this will adversely impact upon the risk management plan and will effectively mean it needs to be rewritten to take this into account.

Defining the risk

The identification of risk is not an easy task and will always be open to interpretation, even between the person being assessed and the assessor, with whom information has been shared. Thus the patient may have a particular perspective about the risks they are facing, some of which is shared by the assessor. However, you may have taken the view that the level of risk is either greater than the person sees it or that there are elements of her/his potential behaviour that pose risks with which they cannot identify (see Figure 3.2).

Johari's Window (Luft and Ingham 1955) postulates that there are aspects of our personality known only to us, as individuals, some which we share with others, some about which we have no insight but which are known to others, and others still that are entirely unknown.

Adapting this model to think about risk, the assessor faces some obvious challenges from the outset. Even if the person being assessed is forthcoming, there are likely to be some elements of risk about which the person will have limited or no understanding. While it may be relatively straightforward to discuss those aspects of risk that the patient can recognise, discussing the elements currently unknown will inevitably be difficult.

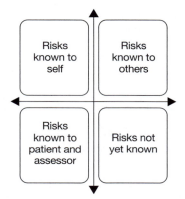

Figure 3.2 Johari's Window adapted for risk (Luft and Ingham 1955)

For example, someone may understand the seriousness of their ideas to harm themselves but have no insight into behaviours that precipitate the risk or place them at risk in other ways. For example, a woman drinking and using illicit substances may not see how that leaves her sexually vulnerable or a person with psychotic phenomena may not link increased illicit substance misuse with an increase in their paranoia and subsequent violence.

Equally, the element of 'unknown to self and others' can act as a useful reminder that, even if you have addressed the risks previously unknown to the person, there may still be risk behaviours, or responses to situations, that neither the assessor or person being assessed have access to, which is what ultimately makes it so difficult to predict. This can only be addressed by asking the 'What if…?' question (see 'What if…? scenario planning' below).

It is worth remembering that identifying risk, or picking out risk factors, only provides information about the risks to then be assessed. That is completed when the likelihood and consequences of the person acting have been worked through and leads to the risk management plan.

What if...? scenario planning

'What if...?' relates to scenario planning. Essentially, it is asking the question: does the person have, or is the person likely to develop, a 'Plan B' if s/he cannot carry out their original plan?

Inevitably, there is a degree of trying to make 'predictions' here but a lot of scenario planning will come from what has happened in the person's past, particularly exploring the detail of past patterns and known risk factors. Going beyond that, thinking about that area where risks are currently unknown to patient and assessor, involves reasoned clinical judgement (Maden 2007; Webster *et al.* 1997). Below are some scenarios to illustrate this.

Scenario 1: If William is harming himself, e.g. cutting his arms when he feels very tense and distressed, if an intervention is put in place to stop him doing this, such as admitting him into hospital, how will he react? The act of bringing him into a different environment may help him feel calmer and more in control. But what if it doesn't and he not only remains prone to feeling tense and distressed but there is nothing in place to help him cope with this, until he starts to feel overwhelmed? Is there a risk that he may now try to harm himself even more seriously or kill himself by using something, e.g. as a ligature?

Scenario 2: If William has been admitted to hospital because he tried to kill himself and this actually increases his feeling of hopelessness, being trapped and unable to think of any other way out of the situation, how will he react? Is there now a risk of him attempting to escape from the ward? If he is to have any leave, how likely is he to abscond if he is with someone or not to return if he goes on his own? Is there even a risk that William may be violent in order to make good an escape, e.g. assault someone then go?

Scenario 3: If William was admitted to hospital because he wanted to kill himself by ingesting prescribed and bought medicines but had ruled out any other method of suicide, might he re-evaluate that when confined to a ward? Is there now a risk of him doing something like attempting to hang himself on the ward, using a plastic bag, or breaking some glass and cutting himself?

Scenario 4: If Michael is more likely to be violent in the context of his delusional beliefs, i.e. thinking people are infecting him, how might this change if he stops taking his medication? If the change is very rapid, might this have to be factored into any leave plan to consider the implications of him absconding and being without prescribed medication for even a short time?

Scenario 5: As with scenarios 1–3, if violence has, effectively, been a maladaptive coping mechanism in the community how will Michael react when in an inpatient environment? Will an acute ward be sufficiently containing or may he need a psychiatric intensive care unit? Equally, if illicit substances have been part of his coping strategy, how will he react without them in a ward environment? How will this impact on the risk of him having drugs smuggled in, absconding, trying to escape or becoming more violent without them?

Scenario 6: Even with an apparently robust plan in place, what if the unexpected happens (see Clinical example 21)? Someone with whom you are managing risk in the community is in a completely uncontrolled environment. Who might they see that could change the risk(s)? What might they do, e.g. use illicit substances, get drunk etc., that would leave them in a disinhibited state and more likely to act in a dangerous way? What could happen to them that would increase their stress, sense of feeling overwhelmed? Importantly, how would they react to the change? Would they be likely to seek help or withdraw from services?

Key to this type of 'What if…?' or scenario planning is that the team, having considered potential risks, now has to incorporate something into the risk management plan to try to prevent it happening. Suddenly the problem is not that the person *was* suicidal but has now been admitted. He *is* suicidal and interventions have to be in place to address this.

Considering potential risks involves exploring an adapted form of the issues listed in section 2 of Part 1 of the *Pocket Guide*, which are:

Early warning signs
How might we know the situation is building towards the person acting in a dangerous way?

What is the person likely to do?
If there was to be a violent act towards others, what, specifically, is it likely to be and is there anyone specifically at risk? If the risk is to self, might it be self-harm or suicide? Might more than one person be at risk?

Motivation and intent
Why would the person act? What would s/he want to achieve?

Severity
What would the likely consequences of the act be? Could it be life-threatening?

Immediacy
Is the person likely to act as soon as s/he had an opportunity? Would certain things have to happen first?

Frequency
Is this something that would be limited to a 'one-off' act? If the person were thwarted, would s/he try again? How quickly? If self-harm or violence, is it likely to be repetitive?

Duration
Are these risk behaviours likely to be present for a long time or are they related to specific events and, therefore, time-limited? If they are related to specific events, are those events likely to recur and, if they do, will they increase the risk again? Equally, are the potential stressors of a more chronic nature e.g. poor interpersonal relationships, and therefore likely to create a constantly volatile environment in which the person is trying to maintain her/his safety?

Likelihood
Ultimately, perhaps the most difficult question is: how likely is it these risk behaviours will actually happen?

Considering how to manage actual and potential risks is detailed in Part 4 but needs to incorporate the following range of issues (see Table 3.5).

Table 3.5 Questions to address potential risk and assist in scenario planning

1. What might make it more likely the person will act?
2. What might make it less likely the person will act?
3. How would you, as a clinician, know, i.e. what is your contact with the person?
4. Has something happened that means you need to re-assess the risk (see Box 6)?
5. What treatment(s) and specific interventions are in place to address and reduce the potential risk behaviours identified?
6. If there are specific individuals at risk, as well as the patient, what is needed to protect them?
7. Are you going to act now or do you need to act if certain circumstances change (again, this brings you back to point 4)?
8. How frequently do you, with the clinical team, need to review the situation (as opposed to carrying out a re-assessment of the patient)?
9. Where does this case sit within your overall clinical priorities? How concerned are you about this person? Have you put sufficient resources and time into safely managing it?
10. Finally, is the person currently in the right environment for you to safely manage the potential risk behaviours with her/him?

Key clinical tip

Think about gaps in your knowledge and understanding of the patient and potential risks. Why is something unclear? Is the patient withholding something, is it unclear to her/himself or have you not asked the right questions or explored things in sufficient depth? Crucially, think of a strategy that will get you the information you need.

Risk to others

If it is established, or you suspect, the person is a risk to others, very specific issues need to be clarified. To do this will involve 'funnelling in':

Clinical example 22: Probing risk to others

Clinician: You said that you still have ideas about harming other people. Is there someone specific you think about harming?

Michael: Did I?

Clinician: Yes. You had mentioned having had thoughts about Daniel and some of the nurses. I wondered if you were still thinking about them.

Michael: Yeah. Yeah, sometimes.

Clinician: You still think about harming Daniel?

Michael: Yeah, but only sometimes.

Clinician: And which nurses do you think about?

Person: Why do you want to know?

Clinician: Because I'm worried about you and what might happen if you do try and harm someone [*pause*]. Can you tell me who it is?

Michael: Ola. And Jane.

Clinician: Is there anyone else?

Michael: No.

Clinician: Are you thinking about harming them now?

Michael: What? Right now? No.

Clinician: But what about today or the last couple of days?

Michael: Yeah. I was thinking about it this morning. When Jane was looking at me. And yesterday when she and Ola were talking about me. What right have they got to do that?

Clinician: And this is about what you fear they might do to you?

Michael: Yeah, messing up my head and all that stuff. That's what they were talking about. And I saw them laughing in the office. They write stuff down about me. In their computers. That goes up on the internet so everyone can read it and it's all lies.

Clinician: Lots of us write things about you, Michael.

Michael: You know what I mean. Not like them.

Clinician: OK. That's interesting. How do you know which of us isn't writing stuff about you, or trying to infect you?

Michael: There's loads of things. The way people stand. The way they look at me, the expression on their face, talk. I just know.

Clinician: You absolutely know?

Michael: Yeah. 'Course I do.

Clinician: What about me, for instance?

Michael: You've always been all right. I've always liked you. Not like them and the stuff they do. It's vile.

Clinician: What might you do about it?

Michael: I don't know.

Clinician: What do you think about doing?

Michael: I told you, I don't know. I might hit them.

Clinician: Have you thought about using a weapon?

Michael: Haven't thought about it.

Clinician: It might be hard to say, but do you think something might happen and you would 'snap', you know, do something without planning?

Michael: Maybe.

Clinician: Have you thought about how you might try and hurt them though?

Michael: I'd only do it because I had to.

Clinician: And what would you do?

Michael: I'd wait 'til they were on their own and maybe use hot water, out of the boiler. That would make them stop.

Here, the clinician keeps returning to the question of who is at risk and, particularly, what Michael might do, as well as what might prompt him to act. Ultimately, she establishes that he would be more likely to carry out a thought through and very violent attack, even if that might ultimately be prompted by something that would make it appear more spontaneous. Michael also gives a clear picture of the effect of his delusional beliefs without ever being asked any direct questions about them. Simply by letting him talk about his beliefs, the full extent of them emerges, as well as some of his reasoning, e.g. who is trying to 'infect him' and how he knows. Unlike in Clinical example 11, when the clinician had to rescue the situation after Michael assumed she didn't believe him because of her choice of words, she is careful to ask about how he knows which of the staff aren't trying to do things to him, thus making it easier to explore without the risk of alienating him. She even feels confident enough to ask him how he feels about her, given the rapport they have established.

Given the psychotic nature of Michael's presentation and the way in which he clearly misinterprets others' actions, knowing exactly what someone may do that would prompt an attack is far more difficult.[1] However, this does not mean an attack is unpredictable. In fact, it is completely predictable, in that it is very likely to happen unless preventative action is taken. Given the biggest causal factor is Michael's psychosis, and that this is most likely to increase when he is very stressed and/or psychologically aroused, actively treating that while at the same time minimising the amount of stress and stimulation he experiences must be a key part of the risk management plan.

At the same time, decisions have to be made about whether or not Michael needs to be moved elsewhere (This would probably be self-defeating as he is likely to develop similar suspicions about others wherever he goes and which may reinforce his paranoia) and whether to move Daniel, Ola and Jane for their own protection. It may be possible to keep them all on the ward together, with a very carefully worked-out plan, but this would rely on having sufficient staff on duty, being able to know the whereabouts of all concerned and the means to evaluate Michael's safety on an ongoing basis.

To summarise, in fully assessing risk to others, as much information as possible is required, including:

* what thoughts the person has about harming others;
* who, if anyone specific, the person is thinking about harming;
* how they might harm the person, e.g. would they use a weapon and if so, what;
* in what circumstances they might harm the person;
* what might stop the person acting upon their thoughts.

If there has been violence
* Why now?
* What were the precipitants?
* Were there specific mental health-related issues?
* Was the person the main perpetrator or did s/he become involved due to the influence of another?

- Did s/he encourage anyone else's participation?
- Was it premeditated or impulsive?
- If it was premeditated, how much planning was involved?
- Were there threats beforehand?
- What stopped the violence, e.g. did the person stop of her/his own volition or due to external causes?
- Did the person have to be physically stopped from continuing the assault?
- If a weapon was used, was it habitually carried or used for that specific assault?
- Was the violence controlled or was there a loss of control?
- Was there any element of sadism, e.g. was there any element of torture or attempt to dominate?

The biggest predictor of future violence is a history of violence, followed by intent, feasibility and capacity (or lack of it). In many cases where you are assessing someone's violence, it will be necessary to get a corroborating account given the likelihood that the person being assessed will minimise the event. Substance misuse and certain personality disorders as well as, to a lesser extent, psychosis will also increase the likelihood of violence (Maden 2007, 2013).

After the violence
- What did the person do afterwards?
- Did s/he admit to the violence or deny it?
- To whom/what does the person attribute responsibility, e.g. the victim, co-perpetrators, circumstances etc.?
- What is the person's attitude towards the violence now?

If someone specific is at risk
- Does that person know?
- Who will notify them?
- Do the police need to be informed?
- It is also important to identify the nature of the violence the person is planning or contemplating, e.g. have weapons been used or are they likely to be?
- If it emerges that the person has used/uses weapons, might they have one with them now and are you safe to continue the assessment?

Key clinical tip

Detail is absolutely crucial in assessing risk to others, as with all elements of risk assessment. The more information about the potential risk, the more robust the risk management plan can be.

Dealing with weapons

If someone has a weapon, you should follow your local policy on how to deal safely with this situation. If your team does not have one, that should be addressed as soon as possible (see also 'Establishing a rapport – skills needed', page 63).

A safety-first approach is *essential*. Unless you are extremely confident you can safely remove the weapon from the setting, you should remove yourself. However, even this is not without risk and simply 'running away', which might be your initial thought, is rarely an option unless you are directly confronted and have no other choice. In part, your decision will be guided by how physiologically aroused the person appears to be – but remember, someone who is outwardly perfectly calm might still be preparing to attack. You may need to address it by direct questions, e.g:

- Do you have a weapon with you now?
- What do you have?
- Where is it?

If it is in a bag or not on the person, e.g. somewhere in the room, you can ask if you can remove it. If you do so, you'll need to hand it to a colleague if in a hospital or clinic setting. If at home, you would need to know it was in another room that the person agrees s/he will not access (remembering that people's homes have numerous things that could be used as a weapon) but should terminate the interview and leave at the earliest possible moment.

Should the weapon be with the person and they want to give it to you, ask that it be placed in a neutral area of the room, e.g. on the table and then take it from there. Do not allow the person to hand it to you directly.

If you suspect a person has a weapon but they either deny this or will not allow it to be removed, you should quietly but firmly terminate the interview and withdraw immediately, seeking assistance.

Key clinical tip

If you have any concerns about a person having a weapon before commencing an assessment – don't. Either have the weapon removed or involve the police immediately. If you begin to suspect the person has a weapon, address the issue and either remove the weapon if safe to do so or terminate the interview and seek assistance.

Risk to self
- Is it suicide?
- Is it self-harm?

Key clinical tip

It is important to remember self-harm and suicide are not the same thing – self-harm can be used as a means to deflect suicidal ideation but people who self-harm can go on to kill themselves either accidentally or intentionally.

Intent
It is crucial to be careful to assess the intent of someone who has either self-harmed or attempted suicide as the nature and consequences of an actual attempt may not mirror the person's intent.

For example, the person may have taken an overdose of a relatively harmless anti-depressant believing it would be lethal. Equally, someone may have taken 30 paracetamol tablets in the belief it would 'put me to sleep for a few days' but not cause any long-term physical harm or actually kill them.

Therefore, explore the detail:

- What did the person want to achieve by their actions, e.g. did s/he intend to kill her/himself?
- Did s/he want to escape her/his situation?
- Did s/he find her/his feelings intolerable and self-harmed or attempted to kill her/himself as it was the only apparent way out of the situation?
- If the person wanted to die, how does s/he feel now, having survived?
- Crucially, having survived, would s/he want to try again – and, if not, why not? What has changed?

The act itself

As with risk to others, explore:

- Why now?
- What protective factors had prevented it until now?
- What were the precipitants?
- Were there specific mental health-related issues?
- Were alcohol or illicit substances a factor?
- Was it premeditated or impulsive?
- If it was premeditated, how much planning was involved?
- Were there 'warnings' or did the person tell anyone beforehand?
- What stopped her/him from continuing the act of self-harm, e.g. did the person stop of her/his own volition or due to external causes?
- Were the means used, e.g. tablets, acquired for this specific attempt?
- How did the self-harm/attempted suicide come to light?
    - Was the person discovered by accident?
    - Did s/he seek help?
    - Did s/he attempt to cover it up or deny it?

After the event:

- What did the person do afterwards?
- Did s/he contact anyone or deny it?
- How was s/he discovered?
- To whom/what does the person attribute responsibility, e.g. self, others, circumstances etc.?
- What is the person's attitude towards the attempt now?

Motivation

Crucially, as you begin to think about developing a risk management plan, the motivation of the person being assessed needs to be considered. Questions that you have to be clear about in your own mind are:

- What does the person see as the problem s/he wishes to address (as opposed to the problem clinicians and/or others are seeking to resolve)?
- What does the person want to achieve now?
- How engaged is s/he in working with you to remain safe?
- Does your risk management plan correlate with the person's level of collaboration (see Figure 3.1).

If the problem the person is grappling with is that s/he finds life unbearable and we are concerned with finding her/him accommodation there is an obvious discrepancy. If we want the person to maintain her/his safety but s/he wants to be dead, that has to be figured into our plan, as we certainly can't rely on that person to do 'what we want'.

When is the person at risk?

- Now?
- If the risk is immediate, is there a risk management plan already in place?
- At some stage in the future what would happen to either increase or decrease the risk?
- Can the person be allowed to leave should they express a wish to do so?

If the person acknowledges they were at risk but no longer are, the key question is, 'What has changed?'. You need to be able to satisfy yourself about what, exactly, has changed for the person that now means they say they can behave in a safe manner.

Moreover, you need to feel satisfied that this is a credible account. It is entirely natural to compose a narrative, retrospectively, to explain to ourselves why we did something or how a series of events occurred. This can vary as time goes on and is more likely to be altered to fit within our overall cognitive schema as we have more time to reflect. It can also feel very difficult for someone to have to tell a relative stranger about something that s/he now finds very embarrassing. Therefore it is important as a clinician to be clear the person is providing an accurate account of events, including their current vulnerability.

The person may have managed to reconstruct their motivation behind the event, as well as how they were feeling, and convinced her/himself it was, for example, something trivial and want to believe they are now 'OK' contrary to the available evidence.

Other factors to consider are that, now the person has acted, s/he feels less aroused and the suicidal impulse has reduced. This may offer you the opportunity to work with someone quite fruitfully but, if there is any ongoing denial of what happened, it is less likely. There is also the risk that any feeling the person has of feeling 'better' will be boosted by being out of the environment and/or situation which precipitated the act, which may contribute to a sense of being able to cope. All of this has to be built into a line of questioning that explores future coping and 'What if?' scenario planning (see 'Defining the risk', page 110).

Finally, you do have to consider whether or not the person is simply lying to you in the hope that s/he will be able to go away and make a further attempt to kill her/himself.

Unless you are convinced something has happened to lessen the risk you should regard it as ongoing.

Where is the person at risk?
- In the department/unit?
- At home?
- What would happen if the person were somewhere else?
- If left alone/unsupported, e.g. without social support, how would this change the risk?
- If a risk to others, is there a context, e.g. might the person be safe with – or away from – another family member?

Why is the person at risk?
There can be numerous reasons the person may be at risk. These vary from the external, e.g. what is happening around them or what others are doing, to the internal, e.g. to their own thoughts and feelings or, more likely, combinations of both. Considering these factors can help with thinking about the likely effectiveness of any proposed risk management plan. Below are three different reasons William might feel suicidal. Each would demand a different clinical response for his safe risk management.

1   Internal

If William is able to identify that he feels suicidal because he cannot bear his feelings, e.g. of loneliness, rejection, loss since Kelly left, he is identifying an internal cause for his behaviour, i.e. his suicidal thoughts have originated from these feelings. In this case, the clinician can begin to explore William's existing psychological and emotional coping mechanisms or previous ways in which he has coped with such difficult experiences and feelings, aiming to build upon these.

2   External

If William tries to kill himself because he wants Kelly to come back, he views the cause as getting Kelly to return. This begs the question of how he will cope if she doesn't return. Since the clinician cannot get Kelly to return, the risk management plan has to take account of his apparent lack of coping mechanisms in her absence. Nor can the clinician rely on tapping into William's coping mechanisms, as he sees the problem – and locus of control – as being external to him. This will increase the risk of further acts of self-harm and/or suicide attempts.

3   Psychotic

If William were to attempt to kill himself because of command hallucinations that have started or worsened since Kelly left and which he cannot resist, the clinician has to immediately address the psychosis as well as William's cognitive and emotional response to her leaving. Key questions would include:

- When did William begin experiencing command hallucinations?
- How severe are they?
- How frequent?
- What does he actually hear?
- Are there times they are worse or better?
- Is anything significant happening at the time?
- Does he hear a variety of commands?
- Are there some he can resist and others he cannot?
- What is he able to do to stop himself acting upon the commands?

Note: it may be that a patient reports acting upon command hallucinations but that these are currently relatively safe. It is crucial to explore what might happen if the commands became more dangerous and plan for such a contingency. There will also be a wide range of factors beyond William's control, such as external stressors that may exacerbate the auditory hallucinations. The risks here are extremely serious.

A recognised assessment tool for exploring psychosis would be useful for an in-depth assessment but may not be practical when conducting a risk assessment. Nonetheless, its absence should not delay the risk assessment.

Other questions to explore when considering why the person is at risk include:

- Is there a pattern?
- Is there a risk profile?
- Do certain events or responses exacerbate or minimise the situation?
- What are the warning signs? Does the person know when things are getting worse and when s/he feels more at risk? How would others, including those caring for her/him, know?

Another aspect of the assessment to consider includes less obvious factors that will impact upon many people who self-harm or act dangerously. These include:

- poor negotiating skills;
- poor problem-solving;
- susceptibility to stress;
- lack of assertiveness;
- lack of social skills;
- peer influence.

The prevalence and severity of these factors need to be taken into account when thinking about risk management (McGranaghan 2004).

Impulsivity

Suicide rarely, if ever, occurs without prior thought or planning. However, some people who survive a suicide attempt will describe the final decision to act as an impulsive phenomenon, a sudden response to a particular trigger that sets in motion the taking of tablets or cutting or going to a physical place to end their life (see, for example, www.kevinhinesstory.com).

This impulse can be transient. If support is available close to or at the moment of impulse, there is the possibility the crisis may be defused. This can be seen at prominent bridges or sites that have seen regular occurrences of suicides. The erection of barriers or placing of nets will stop the person jumping and there is no evidence, i.e. an increase in deaths at nearby bridges, that people immediately look for another opportunity to kill themselves. Moreover, only 5 per cent who were stopped from jumping off the Golden Gate Bridge in San Francisco went on to commit suicide (Guthmann 2005).

Therefore, it is essential to assess how impulsive someone is likely to be, especially because although the action may be impulsive, the person usually has a plan in place that could be lethal.

Another element to impulsivity is the risk of 'opportunistic' self-harm. The person may act upon ideas already formed but not worked into a developed plan because the opportunity presents itself at a time of high arousal.

Groups at most risk of impulsive, dangerous acts include those using alcohol and/or illicit substances, and adolescents.

Rigidity
When feeling suicidal, people are usually constricted in their thinking, mood and action. Their reasoning is dichotomised and, in exploring possible alternatives to death with the suicidal patient, the clinician has to aim to help the person realise there are other options, even if they don't seem ideal.

Short assessments and re-assessments – the key principles

As stated earlier, one of the key principles to an effective risk assessment is devoting the necessary time to it. However, there will inevitably be occasions when the clinician is under pressure to make a brief assessment. Equally, a comprehensive assessment may have taken place in the recent past but there is now a need to re-assess.

The key components for a rapid assessment are:

- The history of the presenting complaint, i.e. what has happened to prompt this presentation and why is it significant now?
- How do these events fit into the person's life?

- A brief overview of the person's history, e.g. family tree, important relationships and life events;
- A summation of her/his current social situation, e.g:
    - What sort of accommodation does the person have?
    - Is s/he working?
    - What social support is available?
    - Has s/he any debts? etc
- Relevant medical and psychiatric history;
- Forensic history;
- Current drug and alcohol use;
- Current mental state examination;
- Risk (to include information highlighted in the introduction, i.e. who, what, when, why and how), as well as:
    - recentness;
    - immediacy;
    - severity;
    - patterns;
    - intent;
    - frequency;
    - plan;
    - level of collaboration;
    - warning signs;
- Formulation – what's happening and why;
- Risk management plan (Harrison and Hart 2006).

Re-assessment should be seen as a routine part of the risk assessment and risk management cycle, particularly given the recognition of risk as a dynamic process. It is always important to remember that it is not just about the individual and her/his own mental, emotional and psychological state, attitudes and behaviour. The context and situation in which the individual is functioning needs constant attention and consideration, as these external factors can have a profound affect on risk (see Box 6). The crucial thing to explore is what has changed since the last assessment and whether or not this increases any previously identified risks or leads to consideration of new risk.

Box 6: Occurrences that should prompt a re-assessment of risk

These would include:

- when a clinician or clinical team receive a referral of a person previously unknown to the service;
- when a person is transferred into a new team or service;
- before and after going on leave;
- following a serious incident or an event that changes the context in which risk behaviours may occur;
- in anticipation of events that are known to increase risk, e.g. bereavement, significant change in relationships etc.;
- before and after any significant change in treatment and/or the patient's management;
- at every Mental Health Act assessment and when considering discharging a patient from a section of the Act;
- prior to discharge from hospital or a community service and, for community services, upon working with a newly discharged patient.

Developing a formulation

This was discussed briefly in the 'Translating the assessment into a formulation' section of Part 2 (page 51). In developing a formulation, you need to consider:

- presenting problems;
- predisposing factors;
- precipitating factors;
- perpetuating factors;
- protective factors;
- underpinning mechanism – the psychological processes and how these produce the presenting problems;
- obstacles to treatment;
- what might stop the person engaging in treatment.

(Adapted from Slesser 2010)

The analysis of these different factors should then lead to a formulation (see Table 3.6).

Following on from an assessment, a formulation helps the clinician – and, therefore, the patient – conceptualise the patient's experience in terms of:

1. What has happened;
2. Who is affected by the event(s);
3. How it has happened;
4. Where it happened and;
5. Why it has happened.

In the case of William, a patient who has attempted suicide and is still experiencing suicidal ideation, this might be written as follows:

> William is a 35 year old, socially isolated and unemployed man currently on Ward X, experiencing suicidal ideation, with a plan to take a further overdose of potentially lethal tablets. He has already ingested approximately 25 paracetamol tablets with the intention of killing himself in the context of poor coping strategies, a traumatic separation from his partner two weeks ago, the anniversary of a significant bereavement and depressive features.

Table 3.6 Formulating the risk

Who is at risk?	William
What is the risk?	Ingested an overdose of paracetamol tablets and still experiencing suicidal ideation
When is William at risk?	Now (currently)
Why is William at risk?	Poor resilience; his emotional and psychological reaction to separation from his wife; and strong depressive features following the death of his father, financial worries and the potential loss of his accommodation. He is unable to access his usual coping strategies and there is an absence of current protective factors in the form of his relationship with his brother and mother
How is William now at risk?	Taking a further overdose

The importance of this structural approach following the identification of risk is that it then makes it easier to develop a risk management plan to address these elements (see Part 4). At the end of the process the clinician should have as clear as possible an idea of:

- how the risk might become acute and/or triggered;
- precipitating, predisposing and perpetuating factors;
- how these factors interact to produce risk.

(Department of Health 2007)

This should all be documented and linked to the risk management plan.

References and selected bibliography

Aldridge, D. (1997) *Suicide: The Tragedy of Hopelessness*. London: Jessica Kingsley.

Appleby, L., Shaw, J., Kapur, N., Windfuhr, K., Ashton, A., Swinson, N. and While, D. (2006) *Avoidable Deaths: Five Year Report by the National Confidential Inquiry into Suicide and Homicide By People with Mental Illness*. Manchester: University of Manchester.

Barker, P. (2003) 'Assessment in practice', in Barker, P. (ed.) *Psychiatric and Mental Health Nursing: The Craft of Caring*. London: Hodder Arnold.

Beck, A. T., Steer, R.A., Beck, J.S. and Newman, C.F. (1993) 'Hopelessness, depression, suicidal ideation and clinical diagnosis of depression', *Suicide and Life Threatening Behaviour*, 23: 139–45.

Casement, P. (1985) *On Learning From the Patient*. London: Routledge.

Colley, G. (2009) *Building Rapport – Customer Relations*. www.evancarmichael.com (accessed 25 January 2011).

Cutcliffe, J.R. and Stevenson, C. (2007) *Care of the Suicidal Person*. London: Churchill Livingston Elsevier.

Department of Health (2004) *The Ten Essential Shared Capabilities*. London: The Stationery Office.

Department of Health (2007) *Best Practice in Managing Risk: Principles and Evidence for Best Practice in the Assessment and Management of Risk to Self and Others in Mental Health Services*. London: Department of Health.

Gladwell, M. (2005) *Blink: The power of Thinking without Thinking*. London: Penguin.

Goleman, D. (1996) *Working with Emotional Intelligence*. London: Bloomsbury.

Guthmann, E. (2005) 'The Allure: Beauty and an easy route to death have long made the Golden Gate Bridge a magnet for suicides', *The San Francisco Globe*.

Harrison, A. (2006) 'Self-harm and suicide prevention', in Harrison, A. and Hart, C. (eds) *Mental Health Care for Nurses: Applying Mental Health Skills in the General Hospital*. Oxford: Blackwell.

Harrison, A. and Hart, C. (eds) (2006) *Mental Health Care for Nurses: Applying Mental Health Skills in the General Hospital*. Oxford: Blackwell.

Hawton, K., Harriss, L. and Zahl, D. (2006) 'Deaths from all causes in a long term follow up study of 11,583 deliberate self harm patients', *Psychological Medicine*, 36: 397–405.

Hoffman, W. and Wilson, T.D. (2010) 'Consciousness, introspection, and the adaptive unconscious', in Gawronski, B. and Payne, B.K. (eds) *Handbook of Implicit Social Cognition: Measurement, Theory, and Applications*. New York: Guilford Press.

Hucker, S. J. (2005) *Psychiatric Aspects of Risk Assessment*. Accessed from: http://www.forensicpsychiatry.ca/risk/assessment.htm

Kingdom, D. and Finn, M. (2006) *Tackling Mental Health Crisis*. London: Routledge.

Kukyen, W. (2006) 'Research and evidence base in case formulation', in Tarrier, N. (ed.) *Case Formulation in Cognitive Behaviour Therapy: The Treatment of Challenging and Complex Clinical Cases*. London: Routledge.

Linehan, M. (1993) *Cognitive-Behavioural Treatment of Borderline Personality Disorder*. New York: Guilford Press.

Luft, J. and Ingham, H. (1955) 'The Johari window, a graphic model of interpersonal awareness', *Proceedings of the Western Training Laboratory in Group Development*, Los Angeles: UCLA.

McGranaghan, T. (2004) *Treatment Risk Information System*. Unpublished paper.

Maden, T. (2007) *Treating Violence: A Guide to Risk Management in Mental Health*. Oxford: Oxford University Press.

Maden, T. (2013) Filmed interview by Justin O'Brien. Unreleased.

O'Brien, J. and Hart, C. (2013) *Clinical Risk Assessment and Risk Management*. London: South West London and St George's Mental Health NHS Trust.

Reynolds, B. (2003) 'Developing therapeutic one-to-one relationships', in Barker, P. (ed.) *Psychiatric and Mental Health Nursing: The Craft of Caring*. London: Hodder Arnold.

Slesser, M. (2010) *Risk Assessment.* http://www.slideserve.com/robbin/risk-formulation (accessed 7 January 2013).

Stuart, G. (2005) 'Therapeutic nurse-patient relationship', in Stuart, G. and Laraira, M. (eds) *The Principles and Practice of Psychiatric Nursing*. St Louis: Elsevier Mosby.

Webster, C.D., Douglas, K.S., Eaves, D. and Hart, S.D. (1997) *HCR-20. Assessing Risk for Violence, Version 2*. Vancouver: Mental Health, Law and Policy Institute, Simon Fraser University.

Wilson, T. (2002) *Strangers To Ourselves: Discovering the Adaptive Consciousness*. Mass.: Harvard University Press.

Note

1   There may, however, be some reality at the root of some of Michael's ideas. He may have a very bad relationship with Daniel and Daniel may, indeed, be doing real things, e.g. arguing with him, talking about him to other patients in a derogatory manner, trying to intimidate him etc., which is another reason to validate the feelings he has rather than question how he interprets events and what he does in response to them. Equally, there may be issues about the body language of some of the nursing staff, how they stand with patients etc., their facial expression or even attitudes that Michael has incorporated into his psychotic world that have a basis in reality and would need to be addressed with the staff.

Part 4: Managing risk

Introduction

There are, essentially, two basic rules for managing risk. Firstly, hope for the best and plan for the worst (Maden 2007). Secondly, always aim for the least restrictive option when working with patients but balance that with consideration for the safety of the patient and/or others and be prepared to be as restrictive as is necessary.

In this final part of the *Pocket Guide*, we will consider the underlying principles and practice of risk management and the use of the information gathered at assessment, developed into a formulation, to progress to risk management with a goal of risk reduction (see Table 4.1). This involves:

- maximising potentially protective factors;
- minimising exacerbating factors;
- acknowledging potential outcomes – and being clear about the potentially best *and* worst;
- ensuring that clinicians given the responsibility for managing the risk also have the *authority* to manage risks identified, e.g.
    - make clinical decisions, including adjusting the risk management plan in response to – and ideally in anticipation of – dynamic change in relation to the person's risk (which is particularly important in inpatient areas);
    - utilise the necessary resources to safely manage the risk, e.g. using more staff on a shift if there is a clear case for how they will be used and the benefits, allocating more time to a patient being seen in the community etc.;
    - managing the environment around the person as much as is practical.

However, it is important to remind ourselves that not every risk can or should be 'managed'. This should obviously be the case if there is not a mental health component to someone's behaviour, e.g. if someone becomes violent when drunk or having taken illicit substances. However, sometimes clinicians allow themselves to be drawn into trying to 'manage' such situations – very rarely happily or with any success.

Nor does even the best assessment allow you to predict the future. What it does allow is for the clinician to develop a coherent, rational plan to address the most obvious or likely risks as well as those already clearly identified. The concept of positive risk management is discussed in the 'Therapeutic risk-taking or positive risk management' section (page 155).

Mental capacity

An important part of considering how collaborative the person is likely to be involves differentiating between situations where you, as a clinician, believe people are at risk and you cannot reach agreement with the patient about how to work in such a way that everyone remains safe, to situations where the patient has come to a rational conclusion that s/he doesn't agree to what seems to others to be a sensible course of action. We cannot explore in detail here issues of capacity and consent and you should familiarise yourself with local and national guidance and policy in this area.

The Mental Capacity Act (2005), Section 2(1) emphasises that healthcare professionals should assume people 16 years old and over are competent to make decisions about their care unless there is evidence to the contrary. The Act goes on to state that a person 'lacks capacity in relation to a matter if at the material time he is unable to make a decision for himself in relation to the matter' due to 'impairment' or 'disturbance in the functioning *of the mind* or brain' (my italics).

The essential issues to consider are:

1. Is the person able to understand and retain the information you are giving her/him and the issues being discussed?
2. Can the person weigh up the information and arrive at a decision?
3. Has the person been able to consider all the options available?
4. Does the person understand the implications of the decision and its likely consequences?

Few could ever agree with an argument put forward by an individual that they had the right to kill someone else or feel unable to take any action to stop them doing it. However, clinicians often find the issue of capacity more complex when considering the case of the suicidal patient. There are ethical, professional and moral issues – which are not always assisted by professional codes of practice – that come into play here but, in the assessment process and thinking about the individual's immediate safety, our duty of care should always lead us to provide adequate safeguards which may not concur with the person's wishes, as well as recognising that capacity is a much more fluid concept, more difficult to assess than many would want to accept.

It is useful to have a solid grounding in the ethics of decision-making and the suicidal patient, but this can often feel very distant to the clinician sitting in the room with someone intent on taking their life. It is thus essential to pay close attention to everything the person says, weighing up her/his internal logic against your own, hopefully, more objective view.

For example, the person may be expressing feelings of hopelessness about their future despite some obvious options for treatment and evidence that s/he would benefit from. In addition, they may be saying they find themselves unable to solve the problems they are faced with when there is evidence these would have easily been within their ability to resolve in the recent past. They may also say everyone will be better off if they are dead, when you have already been alerted by relatives who are very concerned for the person. In such circumstances, it would be difficult to argue that the person has the ability to weigh up information and consider all the options available.

Moreover, there is some evidence emerging from neuro-imaging which has revealed brain abnormalities that are different in people experiencing depression and suicidal ideation and those just depressed. Post-mortem studies have also revealed neurobiological dysfunction related to suicide but independent of major depression. There appear to be three characteristics that differentiate people with depression who are suicidal from people with depression who are not:

1. A sensitivity to particular life events reflecting signals of defeat, based on attentional biases ('perceptual popout') leading to an involuntary hypersensitivity to stimuli which the individual perceives signalling 'loser' status.
2. The sense of being 'trapped', related to insufficient capacity to solve problems, commonly of an interpersonal or social nature.
3. The absence of rescue factors, mediated by deficient prospective cognitive processes and leading to feelings of hopelessness (Van Heeringen and Maruia 2003).

This seems to tie in with cognitive theories and research by Williams *et al.* (2005) and others into what lies behind suicidal ideation, which identify several key factors:

1. **Entrapment** – the inability or perceived inability to escape from 'an aversive environment after one has suffered a defeat, loss or humiliation'.
2. **The arrested flight model** – there are three elements to this:
    a. Sensitivity to cues that signal defeat or humiliation. The person may misinterpret even relatively neutral events, such as the expression on others' faces, chance comments, or view minor issues such as making simple mistakes as complete failure;
    b. An 'overwhelming feeling of *needing to escape*; a sense of being *unable to escape*'. This seems to arise from deficits in interpersonal problem-solving as well as over-generalised memory;
    c. The sense that *this state of affairs will continue indefinitely*, which contributes to the feeling of hopelessness so often described by those experiencing suicidal ideation (italics in original) (Williams *et al.* 2005).

Both of these areas of research suggest that, indeed, there are some profound changes in the functioning of the mind, if not the brain as well.

Exploring options for treatment with people who are psychotic, pose a risk to others and lack capacity or are reluctant to accept treatment, Maden (2007) has argued cogently that all aspects of the individual's capacity have to be explored in depth and clinical teams should adopt the maxim of treating when in doubt on the basis that people have the right to be treated and, despite potential difficulties it may create in the relationship with the individual, the safest option is often the wisest. The same principles could be said to apply to the potentially suicidal person.

Ultimately, while aiming at the least restrictive option when considering any risk management plan, you have to be prepared to consider a plan with sufficient restrictions to provide the safest option for a person lacking capacity or unable or unwilling to cooperate and posing a risk to her/himself or others, including the use of the Mental Health Act 1983 (as amended in 2007), restrictive settings such as inpatient wards and even Psychiatric Intensive Care Units (PICU).

Negotiating and writing a care plan for the purposes of risk management

There is often a great deal of confusion about care plans, how they should be written (and by whom), their purpose and how long they should be in place. It needs to be clear that the care plans highlighted in the *Pocket Guide* are not long term or the type that feature in the Care Planning Approach (CPA) documentation. These are short-term, focused on specific risk issues and designed to be evaluated and adapted as a response to small but important changes, in the context of risk either increasing or decreasing. There are specific interventions to be followed by patient and clinical staff.

Strategies or interventions to directly address the risks identified through a formulation should be translated into clear care plans (see Table 4.1).

Different organisations will have their own way of writing care plans, partly determined by their electronic records system and its framework.

It is important to acknowledge that many electronic record systems are far from perfect, particularly in providing a simple pathway from assessment to formulation to care plan. This constitutes a clear organisational risk and should be addressed as soon as possible. Equally, the education of users of these systems is often far from complete and there may be many advantages to the system about which clinicians are unaware.

Clinicians involved in using electronic systems with particular structural frameworks should familiarise themselves with them in as much detail as possible but also be aware of their limitations. They must ensure that this does not impact upon the crucial function of the risk management plan, which is to do as much as possible to ensure the safety of the patient and others by:

1. Identifying potential risks and 'problem behaviours' associated with those risks;
2. Providing a clear objective to meet the problem;
3. Listing the necessary interventions to make it possible to achieve the objective and who will do what for each intervention.

Table 4.1 A framework for a risk management plan.

Clear identification and description of the risk, in the simplest, most easily understandable terms.	Is the risk actual (immediate) or potential, e.g. something will have to happen to increase the risk?
Identify who is at risk, naming the person(s) involved or at risk, e.g. *William wants to kill himself etc.; Michael wants to assault Daniel etc.*	How willing is the person to collaborate: • Will this be a care plan or a management plan?
Name the desired outcome (objective) directly related to the specific problem identified.	If the person is collaborating, the objective would be that s/he will keep her/himself safe. If there is no collaboration it would be that the team will work to keep the person safe.
List the interventions required to achieve the objective.	Maximise potentially protective factors and minimise exacerbating factors.
Who, specifically, will do what to manage the risk?	• The patient; • The primary nurse/keyworker; • Others from the MDT.
A time frame for addressing the situation/behaviours.	This should be short enough to adapt the plan according to whether or not it is working, i.e. a few days only.

Even when someone is feeling very distressed and/or disturbed, it is usually possible to have a conversation about what s/he wants or, preferably, needs to help her/him at that time. As has been stated throughout the *Pocket Guide*, developing a collaborative approach should always be the clinician's goal and this is equally true for care plans.

If, for any reason, the person is unable to work with you to keep her/himself and others safe, this *has* to be pro-actively addressed. It is one of the very few times that you, in collaboration with the rest of the clinical team, should impose a care plan. This will almost always happen in an inpatient environment or PICU and, in such cases, it is important that the ownership of the problem is with the team and, most particularly the ward nurses, as it is the nurses who will spend the majority of time with the person and may have to physically intervene to maintain everyone's safety. Therefore, the interventions should remain with the nurses and other team members but be specific, clear and with the single objective of keeping the person and others safe.

Below are two examples of safety care plans, one for an inpatient setting, one for the community, and a risk management plan for a non-collaborative patient. As well as care plans being shaped by electronic record systems, particular organisations may also have models or templates for the writing of care plans. Nonetheless, it is useful to look at some simple principles that make the plan easy to write, understand and implement, as well as measurable and straightforward to evaluate.

Principles of care planning

The concept of a care plan is to provide the clinician and patient an agreement about:

- what will be discussed:
  - the identification of a clear problem or need;
  - a proposed solution (the objective);
  - the interventions to achieve the solution;
- how often the discussion will take place;
- how long the discussions will last;
- the overall time frame over which the work will take place (Ritter 1989).

It is essential that a safety care plan is about *one* problem or need, which is the identified risk. This should never be conflated with other issues. This is true even when the risk is associated, for example, with psychosis. In an instance like this there should be a care plan for treating the psychosis, e.g. by the administration of medication etc., and a separate plan for addressing the risk issues.

A care plan (as opposed to a management plan that has to be imposed on a patient for safety reasons) should also be:

- recovery oriented;
- person centred and coming from the person's perspective;
- written in simple language and, if not using the person's own words exactly, retaining their spirit while conserving a structure that will enable other clinicians to understand and use the plan in a consistent fashion and for it to be evaluated.

A structure for writing care plans

The starting point has to be a conversation between yourself and the patient. As has been emphasised throughout, the goal of the assessment is to identify any risks affecting the person you are assessing. However, you should also be attempting to do this in such a way that you arrive not only at a shared understanding of those risks but also at potential solutions. A number of clinical examples demonstrate how this can be achieved.

The conversation can then focus on explicitly naming the problem, which allows an equally explicit statement about the solution, or objective. These components of a plan are sometimes easier than working through who will do what, in terms of interventions. However, careful listening to the person will usually offer clues (see Clinical example 23).

Clinical example 23: Negotiating a safety care plan in a community setting

Clinician: I know this has been a very difficult conversation and we've covered a lot of ground, but I'm still wondering about how Jenny and I can help you remain safe.

William: I told you, I'll be OK.

Clinician: I'd like to think that. But you've talked quite a lot about having had these ideas about trying to kill yourself and even how you'd do it. To be honest, that doesn't sound OK to me.

William: [*Silence*]

Clinician: Earlier on, I touched on some ideas…

William: [*Interrupts*] I'm not going into hospital. I told you that.

Clinician: Yes, you did. But my concern is that something might happen and you might end up taking some tablets. I want to discuss some quite specific things to help you keep yourself safe.

William: Do you think I'm still thinking about killing myself or I'd do anything like that after talking with you?

Clinician: [*Pause*] I'm not sure. Do you?

William: [*Long pause*] What about if I come and see you regularly?

Clinician: How would that help, do you think?

William: It's helped me today. I feel like I've cleared my head a bit. [*Pause*] You know, I've also realised maybe I can be helped. I don't know … I felt really helpless, like there was no way out…

Clinician: And now?

William: Well, if I can get some sleep at night, like you said, I'm going to feel better for that. And I can stay with my mum 'til my brother gets back. I don't want to worry her though…

Clinician: But you said she is worried about you.

William: Yeah. Now I wish I'd listened to her and James and tried to get some help earlier. Or even said more to Dr Patterson when I saw her at the surgery.

Clinician: So coming in to talk with me would help. And getting more sleep.

William: Yes.

Clinician: What else? You did mention there were things you used to do when you were feeling down that helped you.

William: You said about making some lists of things that help me and stuff that drags me down. I could do that.

Clinician: Would you be able to do that before you come in to see me next time? [*William nods*] Sometimes it's useful if people also make a note of what helps and what makes things worse, and how that varies during the day.

William: Um, I mentioned some of that stuff, didn't I? Like feeling worse in the evening, when I start thinking a lot about Kelly not being there.

Clinician: Yes, and we did talk about the early evening possibly being a good time to go for a walk…

[*Later in the interview*]

Clinician: OK, while you and Jenny were talking, I've made a note of where we've got to. As I said earlier, we try and write these plans or agreements in a certain way but I've tried to capture what we were talking about. Would you take a look and see what you think?

William: [*Reads the care plan*] Yes, it's OK.

Clinician: The most important thing is, do you think it's manageable for you?

William: Even talking about it now has helped. I don't know. It's given me something to think about and I've got things I can do.

Clinician: So we'll see you tomorrow and we'll also come to see you on Thursday. After that, we'll review whether or not we still need to meet daily.

William: Yeah.

Clinician: And you have our number, in case you need to get in touch in between meeting up.

William: Uh huh.

Clinician: What would you do if you felt you were getting towards that stage where you can't cope and might do something to harm yourself?

William: Well, I'd ring you or come down to the health centre. And if it was at night...

Clinician: Which it might be...

William: Then I'd ring that crisis line number or I could call James.

Clinician: And it's OK for us to ring James and talk with him?

William: I think it would help. You know, even though we're close, it would be difficult for me to tell him some of this stuff straight off.

Clinician: OK that's good. You could go to A&E as well.

William: I told you, I don't want to do that, because I'll end up seeing some doctor I don't know and they'll want to admit me to hospital. Anyway, I've got rid of all the tablets in the house and you'll only be bringing me a day's worth at a time.

Clinician: I want to keep coming to A&E as an option, because at least we'll know you're safe.

William: I'll be honest. I'd have to really be feeling desperate. And, anyway, you said that crisis team could come out if I needed them.

Clinician: Yes, they can, but I have to be honest as well. It can take a while. But, if things start to really get on top of you and you start to feel like you're going 'nuts', as you talked about earlier, you might need to get help right away. That's why I think calling for an ambulance might be necessary. They may even be able to help you with getting the crisis team but, if not, they can take you somewhere safe for a while.

William: [*Silence, then nods*]

Clinician: There's one last thing I need to discuss with you.

William: Look, I'm really tired…

Clinician: I'm sorry. This is important though.

William: OK.

Clinician: Supposing something happens that you're not expecting, like you see Kelly, or you have a terrible night and can't sleep. And you think about giving the team a call but the thought of killing yourself comes back and is stronger than you feel able to cope with?

William: I won't see Kelly. That won't happen.

Clinician: I don't mean intentionally, necessarily. Suppose you just see her in the street?

William: [*Silence*]

Clinician: Would you tell me what you're thinking about?

William: [*Pause*] I was thinking … about what would happen … how I'd feel if I did see Kelly…

Clinician: It's not just that I'm talking about though. I'm talking about something unexpected that throws you off balance and you struggle to cope with. It might be another bill coming in through the post, a phone call, bad news about something. You remember we talked earlier about how people in your situation can find it difficult to solve problems or work their way through situations they normally would, and then you can feel trapped, with no way out?

William: Yeah. I know that feeling only too well.

Clinician: That's why I want to keep something like the A&E option open. You only have to ring 999 and let a paramedic through the door.

William: You worry too much.

Clinician: [*Smiles*]

William: OK. But I don't think I'll need it if you bring me those sleeping tablets. And you were saying the anti-depressants will start working in a few more days.

Clinician: Well, more like a week or so. But it feels like we have got a plan.

William: Yes.

Example of a safety care plan in the community

In this example, following William being referred to the community mental health team by his GP after complaining of anxiety and not sleeping, he has been assessed and the plan touched upon in Clinical example 23 negotiated to help him keep himself safe while remaining in his flat. This is how it might read:

Problem:
Over the last week, I (William) have been thinking about killing myself in my flat.

Objective:
I (William) will keep myself safe for the next three days in my flat and when I'm out.

Interventions
I (William) will:

1. Meet each day, for 45 minutes, with Carol or Jenny to talk about how I'm coping and how safe I feel.
2. Make a list of things that used to help me when I felt depressed and had ideas about harming myself.
3. Make a list of things that make me feel worse and things that make me feel better now.
4. Bring the lists in with me for Wednesday's appointment and discuss them with Carol and Jenny.
5. Go for a 20-minute walk twice a day, once at lunchtime and once in the evening.
6. Get in touch with Mum and James to let them know what I'm doing and ask for help if I need it.
7. Contact Carol or the team if I feel unsafe or am worried that I might harm myself. If it's after the team have finished work, I'll contact the crisis team or ring for an ambulance to take me to A&E.
8. Take the sleeping tablets and anti-depressant tablets as prescribed.

My nurses will:

1. Meet me each day, for 45 minutes, to talk about how I'm coping, how to solve any problems I am having and how safe I feel.
2. Discuss my lists with me and how I can use them to help me stay safe.

3. Get in touch with James to let him know what's been happening and make sure he feels OK to help.
4. Be available to meet me urgently if I feel unsafe or am worried that I might harm myself. Let the crisis team and A&E team know I might need to get in touch in the evening and give them a copy of this care plan.
5. Give my sleeping tablets to me each day.

In the above example, William is an active participant in the care plan process. The clinician, Carol, writes the plan in a way that captures William's words and what he is prepared to do, though she was very assertive with him about keeping the option of using the A&E department open in case of an unforeseen emergency. Whether or not he would use that option is debatable but she has got his agreement on everything else, so is working on the basis of there being sufficient interventions to help William remain safe.

In not admitting him to hospital, there is an element of positive risk-taking but this plan sits clearly within the essential principles of a recovery approach and positive risk management (see 'Therapeutic risk-taking or positive risk management' on page 155), while being practical and clinically sound. The structure of the care plan is detailed in Table 4.2.

Table 4.2 Structuring a care plan

Identifying the problem	Setting an objective to resolve the problem
Concerned person (whose problem is it?)	*Concerned person (who will take responsibility for the solution?)*
William	William
Problem	*Objective*
Has been thinking about killing himself	Will keep himself safe
Context or setting	*Context or setting*
In his flat	In his flat and outside
Time frame(s)	*Time frame*
Over the last week	Over the next three days

The simplicity of the care plan is, hopefully, apparent. It could be followed by anyone if either Carol or Jenny were unavailable and, were William to need to contact the crisis team, it would give a clear indication of the problem and strategies to help William keep himself safe.

The point of having William as the concerned person, both in 'owning' the problem and being responsible for the solution is not just about helping him with his recovery but also because, ultimately, he will be the only person able to keep himself safe, as evidenced by the fact that people manage to self-harm and even kill themselves when in hospital, including when they are being closely observed (Appleby *et al.* 2006).

However, the clinicians are taking a very active role in supporting him with this, with their interventions mostly mirroring his, e.g. meeting with him, looking at his list, helping him problem-solve, calling his brother and giving him his medication on a daily basis initially. All of these things are very directly linked to elements that contribute to his suicidal ideas, as well as allowing them to focus on the specific issues with which he is grappling.[1]

The second example looks at how William's risk management is organised in an inpatient setting, which would take place in a situation where he was only able to provide limited assurances of his ability to keep himself safe.

This does not necessarily mean that he would need to be formally admitted to hospital under a section of the Mental Health Act. The skills used in assessing the person and negotiating options for her/his safety can go a long way in facilitating a plan where the person may agree to things they don't particularly like but can recognise are probably necessary. However, you should always understand the necessity of using more restrictive options when there is no other obvious, safe choice.

Example of a care plan in an inpatient ward
In this example, William didn't go to see his GP, but rang for an ambulance, having actually taken an overdose of 20 paracetamol tablets then feeling panicky and regretful. However, assessed in the A&E department, he was clear he had tried to kill himself and ambivalent about surviving the suicide attempt. He was then admitted to an acute psychiatric ward. This care plan was written after William asked to leave the ward to go and get some clothes from his flat three days after being admitted and was found by the nurse re-assessing him to be experiencing suicidal thoughts again.

Problem:
I [William] currently want to kill myself on the ward.

Objective:
I [William] will stay on the ward for the next three days and not harm myself.

Interventions
I will:

1. Make a list of things I used to do to help myself if I was feeling down or unable to cope.
2. Do one of the things that help me cope to remain safe if I feel unsafe on the ward.
3. Meet with my nurses once a day, for 15 minutes, to look at other things I can do to help me stay safe.
4. Acknowledge the nurse checking my safety every 15 minutes and, if I feel I'm unable to cope or might harm myself, alert the nurse and discuss immediate steps to maintain staying safe.

My nurses will:

1. Make a copy of my list of things I used to do to help myself if I was feeling down or unable to cope.
2. Meet with me each day, for 15 minutes, to discuss other things I can do to help me stay safe.
3. Check my safety every 15 minutes and, if I feel unable to cope or might harm myself, discuss with me immediate steps to maintain my safety.

Again, the principles here are the same: collaborative, recovery oriented and aimed at addressing elements that contribute to his suicidal ideas, as well as allowing them to focus on the specific issues with which he is grappling.

Documentation after a re-assessment of risk

See 'Record-keeping and good documentation' (page 161) for principles about good documentation. The most important thing to remember is that, if it isn't written down, to all intents and purposes, it didn't happen, so recording what you've done with a patient is essential.

In the example below, the clinician is documenting the re-assessment that led to the writing of the above, inpatient care plan:

At approximately 16.20 hrs William asked to leave the ward to get some things from his flat, saying he would return within two hours. I reminded him of his care plan, to stay on the ward, but he was insistent he be allowed to leave. We met for 15 minutes to discuss. Initially, he was reluctant to talk, didn't say what had changed from his earlier distress and, particularly, when he was saying he wanted to die. He said, several times he was 'all right' and not thinking about harming himself.

Through direct questioning about his mental state, William acknowledged he is sleeping poorly, having difficulty getting to sleep and waking early, is ruminating about his break up with Kelly and cannot see anything positive in his future. Concentration and appetite are poor, he is 'not enjoying anything' and, when asked, 'can't see anything good' in the future. Said he felt worse because of noise on the ward, 'being surrounded by mad patients' and an incident on the ward this morning when a patient was restrained.

He became very distressed as he spoke more, but said he has been feeling his 'head will explode' with 'pressure' and needed to leave the ward because he couldn't think and needed to get away from how he was feeling. Although initially denying suicidal thoughts, went on to describe feeling he 'couldn't carry on without Kelly'. Acknowledged he had wanted to die when took previous overdose and now was thinking about taking more tablets when he got home because he needed to 'escape [his] unbearable feelings'.

At end of conversation, agreed to stay. I have changed his current safety care plan and William agreed to the changes, taking away a copy. Same written in progress notes below but also in care plan section of RIO. Risk assessment section updated.

A management plan for a patient who cannot or will not collaborate

As has been noted, there will be times when, despite the efforts of the clinical team, the patient either cannot or will not collaborate. When there are sufficient concerns about specific risks, this necessitates the team initiating a management plan. Below is an example:

Problem

Over the past two days, Michael has made specific threats to harm fellow patient, Daniel, and nurses Ola and Jane on the ward and cannot agree a way in which he can behave safely.

Objective

Over the next three days, the team will try to maintain Michael's and others' safety on the ward.

Team interventions on the ward

1. Have a nurse within sight of Michael at all times, making sure he does not get into physical altercations with other patients or become verbally abusive and threatening. Note – help is to be summoned immediately if Michael becomes verbally abusive or physically threatening, using the alarm if necessary.
2. Ensure Michael is not in the same part of the ward as Daniel or any other patient whose behaviour may inadvertently provoke a potentially aggressive reaction from him.
3. Ola and Jane will not work on the same shift and staff will always know both their and Michael's whereabouts when they are in the ward environment.
4. Help Michael take part in low stimuli activity on the ward and, if he is able, games with members of staff.
5. If Michael is over-stimulated by being with other patients at mealtimes, to have his meals on his own, either separately in the dining room or in his room.
6. Fully re-assess Michael's safety each shift, based on his behaviour, actions towards others and ability to reach agreement with nursing staff. This is to be repeated if specific changes are noted that might increase risk.
7. Give Michael a ten-minute period each shift when he can spend time with the nurse to talk about anything he needs or anything he thinks will help him, encouraging him towards a more collaborative approach.
8. If he becomes very unsettled, quietly talk with him about things that help him feel calm and in control.
9. Administer PRN medication if he asks for it or a decision is made that he needs it.
10. If Michael makes continuing threats to staff or other patients, or hits anyone on the ward, he should be placed in seclusion until it is assessed he will be safe back on the ward.

In this instance, a plan has been put in place by the clinical team because their assessment is that Michael is currently too psychotic to be able to agree a plan that he can consistently implement. Therefore they have put in place a number of clear interventions they will undertake in order to try and keep both him and others safe. Because there are a number of things an incoming shift team would have to be aware of, it would be necessary to have paper copies available to them to read and also to go through it at shift handover.

Although the plan runs for three days before a multi-professional team review, it would be necessary for the nursing staff to review it on a shift by shift basis and adjust it as necessary. For instance, it may be too dangerous to leave the nurses at risk on duty on the ward or Daniel, the patient being threatened, may not be willing to keep moving if Michael wants to be in a certain part of the ward.

The plan makes allowance for every attempt to engage with him and seek his collaboration, as well as any escalation of the risk and a contingency to meet this, i.e. for Michael to be moved into the seclusion facility on the ward.

Should it be necessary to nurse Michael in the seclusion facility, clear criteria should be identified that would be met before he returned to the ward – not just that he is not actively exhibiting any challenging behaviour. This should include a review of Michael's mental state as well as his willingness/ability to cooperate with nurses' requests when they enter the room to talk to him. In Michael's case, the criteria for his return onto the ward might be that he will agree to:

1. Having a nurse with him at all times.
2. To stay away from Daniel, Ola and Jane until it is clearly established he can safely be in the same room.
3. To tell nursing staff how he is feeling, what is helping him feel calm and able to behave safely and what might make him feel like harming someone.
4. To take oral medication, as prescribed.
5. Not to behave in a threatening or dangerous manner, e.g.
    a. not threatening staff or other patients;
    b. not being physically violent to people or damaging property.

From the clinician's perspective, this is about establishing clear boundaries and providing a safe and containing environment. Michael might even be forced to take medication against his will if it is assessed as being necessary. However, he may well experience this as wrongfully being deprived of his liberty, punitive and alienating.

It should also be remembered that this can be terrifying, even for an individual whose outward behaviour is perceived as 'hostile', 'threatening' or even physically 'violent'. This is where the importance of the different components of care becomes apparent. It is also worth remembering at this point that the majority of incidents of violence and aggression from patients seen in psychiatric units are 'defensive' in nature, i.e. result from the patient perceiving themselves to be threatened or in situations in which they feel they are in danger, feel their requests are being deliberately frustrated or nurses are overly and unnecessarily controlling (Breeze and Repper 1998; Hamolia 2005). Carefully communicating what is being done, and why, and using de-escalation skills to try and keep the environment around the patient as calm as possible are essential. In addition to this, a session with a patient who has been in seclusion to help her/him evaluate the experience should always occur (Hart 2013a).

It may take some time to affect improvements in the person's mental state or how s/he perceives what is happening. Certainly, you cannot reassure them that things are 'all right'. Nor will they agree to any attempts you make to get them to 'calm down'. However, you can stabilise many of the things around them. Your calmness, consistency and confidence in what you are doing can be very containing (Casement 1985). You can also affect the environment, minimise the stimulation around them and maintain the physical safety of the patient and others (Hart 2013b).

Inpatient nurses should not shy away from providing these important nursing treatments, and proactively intervening. Indeed, what is often termed (and shaped as) enhanced observation can be re-thought of as enhanced personal support, with the nurse allocated to continuously be with the patient working to a care plan that is geared towards specific risk management interventions rather than nebulous observations, with the nurse allocated often not even sure what s/he is supposed to be observing (Onyenaobiya and Hart 2013). To get to a position where you can introduce a higher level of care can be delicate but usually requires the clinician to be clear, direct and honest (see Clinical example 24).

Clinical example 24: Confronting the person you think is at serious risk

William: Look, are you letting me out of this place or not?

Clinician: I know you're saying that you feel OK now but I can't see what has changed since you took the tablets and wanted to kill yourself.

William: No. I'm OK now.

Clinician: You say that but you still look very low – just as you did when you arrived.

William: Yeah, well, whatever you say, I really want to go and I'm going now.

Clinician: You were saying when we spoke a while ago that you didn't sleep well last night and were feeling very on edge. You know, I'm just worried about you right now and I'd like the chance to talk some more with you about what's difficult about staying here.

William: I'm not talking anymore. I'm going and that's it.

Clinician: I can't change your mind?

William: No.

Clinician: Well, I'm sorry, but I can't just let you leave.

William: Why not?

Clinician: Because I can't see anything that makes me think things are any better for you.

William: Are you calling me a liar?

Clinician: You were saying earlier that things definitely weren't all right. I have a serious concern that, if you had the opportunity, or could see no other way out of your situation, you might try again to kill yourself.

William: That's rubbish. I told you things have changed and I'm going.

Clinician: I am sorry, William, because I don't want to act against your wishes, but in the interests of your safety, I'm going to keep you here and ask a doctor to conduct an assessment under the Mental Health Act of 1983, with a view to detaining you for your own safety.

William: What? You can't do that. You're treating me like a little kid.

Clinician: I know you will find this very difficult but I don't think I have any other choice.

The clinician here is absolutely clear and direct in communication, expressing the exact nature of her concerns, why she has them and what she is doing as a consequence. She recognises and acknowledges both the area of disagreement and the impact it has on the patient, empathises but does not allow his distress to cloud her clinical judgement. When William asks if she is calling him a liar, rather than 'defend' herself or get into a 'yes/no' discussion, she simply reminds him of things he has already said that have led her to her conclusion.

Behaving in a consistent, clear and compassionate fashion, alongside the other communication skills required when having to go against the wishes of the patient in a particularly challenging situation, will do as much as anything to 'contain' the patient's anxiety and assist in trying to maintain a relationship with the patient that has its basis in being helpful, genuine and honest.

Key clinical tip

The five 'Cs' help **contain** the patient's distress when you're going against her/his wishes in exerting your **clinical** judgement in a **challenging** situation.

Communicate in a way that is:

1. consistent;
2. clear;
3. compassionate;
4. concise;
5. caring.

Therapeutic risk-taking or positive risk management

Therapeutic risk-taking or therapeutic risk management has to be separated from taking risks without the clinicians involved having seriously thought about the issues or discussed them with the patient. Therapeutic risk-taking is deciding upon a plan of action that does have recognised associated risks, when the potential benefits outweigh the potential negative consequences of the plan. An example of this might be agreeing with William he will remain in his flat and be seen on a daily basis after he has been assessed, having seriously considered ingesting a number of analgaesia tablets above the prescribed dose while in an emotionally distressed state. The risk is not completely eliminated at this stage but this approach is judged to be more beneficial than admitting him into an acute ward against his will in that it allows him to maintain a degree of manageable responsibility for his safety, assists the team in engaging with him and takes advantage of his collaboration in his risk management. It also means that the potential negative experience of being on a psychiatric ward is avoided.

Positive risk-taking can only take place in the context of a robust risk assessment and risk management plan, taking into account advance directives (where these are in place), and an exploration of 'what if?' scenarios and contingency plans. It is reliant upon having developed, with the patient, a shared understanding of the potential risks to the patient of their own behaviours, and the drivers for these behaviours. It involves balancing the negative consequences of these risk behaviours, were they carried out, with the positive benefits of the use of agreed, adaptive coping mechanisms to combat them. Focusing on the strengths of the patient and their social network, it offers the opportunity for the person to drive her/his own recovery with others' help (see Box 7 below).

Positive risk management should have been agreed within the whole clinical team and the clinician(s) working directly with the patient should also be receiving consistent and regular supervision which allows the opportunity to discuss and reflect on potential decisions that can allow 'reality checks' on what is safe, what is possible and what actual risks are being addressed, and how.

The underlying principles of positive risk management are that clinical decisions should always be defensible rather than defensive, in the best interests of the patient and seeking to provide the least restrictive options in terms of their care. It has to be acknowledged that there are inherent risks in this, e.g. granting someone leave from the ward when they have previously been expressing ideas of self-harm but are now providing assurances of how they can manage these and not act upon them. Other issues to consider are:

- the benefits of admitting someone to hospital against working with them while they remain in their home;
- the level of responsibility someone can take in maintaining their own safety;
- the long-term impact of taking restrictive measures for the immediate safety of the individual and/or others, against the wishes of the person, which might make engagement and the development of a therapeutic alliance far more difficult.

Box 7: A checklist for teams and patients when working with positive risk management

1. Are you clear about the service user's experiences and understanding of risk?
2. Are you clear about the carer experiences and understanding of risk (primarily, are they happy about the particular risks to be taken and any responsibility that may be placed upon them)?
3. Have you clearly defined potential risks and their context?
4. Has there been a clear articulation of the desired outcomes?
5. Has there been a clear identification of strengths and coping mechanisms?
6. Is everyone clear about the planned stages for risk-taking?
7. Has there been an estimate of potential pitfalls and estimated likelihood?
8. What potential safety nets are in place, including identification of early warning signs linked to a crisis and contingency plan?
9. Have you and the patient explored the 'what if' scenarios?
10. What was the outcome of previous attempt(s) at this course of action?
11. How was it managed, and what will now be done differently?
12. What needs to, and can, change?
13. How will progress be monitored?
14. Who agrees to the approach (and who disagrees)?
15. When will it be reviewed?

(O'Brien and Hart 2013)

Relapse profiles and crisis plans

If you and your team have been involved in caring for, and treating, someone who has been through a crisis, it is always useful to evaluate with them what happened during that period and, even more importantly, the events that led up to it. From such a discussion two things can be developed that will be useful in the event of a change in the person's circumstances that could lead to a further crisis. The first is a relapse profile. There are a number of models for this, some involving work with the individual concerned, others that explore relapse prevention and self-monitoring from the perspectives of the patient, family and staff (Gamble and Curthoys 2004). The example below (Box 8) involves looking at the events that occurred, and their impact on the person's mental health.

Box 8: A sample relapse profile

Thoughts	Feelings	Behaviour
I think Kelly is fed up with me because she thinks I'm not a good partner and can't provide for her.	I feel misunderstood and anxious.	I compensate by doing things I think will please Kelly.
This is too hard and I'm not getting anywhere. Kelly's getting at me.	I feel more anxious but also frustrated.	I stay in and do less. I try to avoid Kelly but argue because I think she's angry with me. We stop having any sexual relationship.
I lie awake worrying about things that have happened, especially about my dad's illness and his death, and what may happen next day.	I feel tired and irritable.	I try to communicate how I'm feeling but find myself complaining and arguing even more.

Thoughts	Feelings	Behaviour
Kelly is going to leave me. Things will go wrong. I can't pay my bills. I'm going to lose the flat. I let my dad down. I should have done more.	Abandoned and 'lost' but also alone and resentful. Guilty.	I stop going out, spend more time on my own, staying in bed, not answering the phone.
Others think I can't cope and I'm weak. No one understands or wants me around. People blame me for everything. When I can't sleep, I start to think about harming myself in the early hours.	Really miserable and tired. I don't feel hungry, don't feel like doing anything. Ashamed. I want this to end.	I eat less but start drinking alcohol more than I should. I sleep less and wake up early. Avoiding people and don't want to talk to anyone about how I feel.
There's no solution to my problems. It's all my fault. I'd be better off dead.	I feel trapped, boxed in and have to get away, but I'm not really sure what I want to get away from or where to go.	I withdraw even more and start drinking more and more.
There's only one way out. I have to kill myself. I start thinking of how I will do this.	There's no way to describe how I feel.	If no one stops me or reaches out to me, I will kill myself.

Drawing up something like this with the person is a good way for both of you to understand the process, piece by piece, by which the original crisis came about. In doing this you can also help the person identify warning signs of when things might start to be recurring, or a relapse starting. Even if there are significant changes in the person's experience, as is the case with William, where he has separated from his partner, he can look back on the pattern of his thoughts, how they relate to his feelings and how both affect his behaviour.

As a result of this exercise, which might take a number of sessions to allow the person the opportunity to reflect and help them with some painful feelings, s/he can begin to think about a crisis plan to try to prevent a relapse (Hillard and Zitek 2004). This can be formatted into a plan in much the same way immediate risk management plans are.

Steps to help William prevent a crisis

1. Make sure I eat regularly (and not too late) and get enough sleep.
2. Exercise every day, even if it's just going for regular walks, but preferably attending yoga classes and playing football with my friends.
3. Keep my routine going, even if I'm not working.
4. Set myself daily tasks to do and keep to my plans.
5. Visit my brother and mum once a week, let them know how I'm feeling and get feedback from them about what they see me doing.
6. Start looking for work, but if I can't find anything remind myself that there are about 15 to 20 people looking for every job available.
7. Keep my alcohol intake to no more than two to three pints a week and don't drink spirits.

If I start to become anxious and miserable or thinking about harming myself

1. Check my list of things to prevent a crisis and see if I'm doing everything – if not, try to do it.
2. Challenge any negative thoughts.
3. Check things out with people, e.g. what they're thinking, how they feel towards me.
4. Do routine deep breathing and relaxation exercises four times a day and when I'm starting to feel more anxious than usual.
5. If things get worse, contact the community mental health team and ask for an urgent appointment.
6. If I have an unexpected crisis, ring the crisis helpline or go to the A&E department.

Crisis plans can be very helpful but the more work that goes into addressing the problems that led to the original clinical presentation, the less likelihood there will be of the person relapsing. In that work, the assessment of risk and risk management will be crucial.

Record-keeping and good documentation

Good record-keeping is an integral part of risk management. Anything you write about the risk assessment should be directly relevant to that, as objective as possible, and avoiding labels and terms such as 'angry', 'violent', 'dangerous', which are highly subjective. Instead, you should describe any act that has taken place, e.g. 'Michael was shouting loudly, swearing and making threats to staff. He then threw a chair across the room at Staff Nurse Murray which narrowly missed her legs', or 'Michael shouted at Nurse Murray, saying that he would hit her if she did not leave the room but walked away without any intervention'. If generic terms such as 'anger' or 'violence' are used, the clinician should be as precise and accurate as possible when communicating with others, either orally or in documentation.

It is important to differentiate between fact and opinion. It may be a fact that William took a large number of paracetamol tablets. The intent may not be clear and William may be saying afterwards that he did not intend to kill himself. You should not write down your own ideas about his intentions as if they are fact. Rather, indicate your subjective impression, e.g. 'William took 30 paracetamol tablets last night at approximately 21.00 hrs. Although he now states he did not intend to kill himself, it is my impression that he wanted to die and was disappointed to have survived the self-poisoning. This is based on his brother's account of what he had been saying in the days leading up to the incident and his reluctance to attend the A&E department. It was also noted by A&E nurses that he was tearful and saying he "could not believe he had messed this up".'

It is also important to remember anything you record will be open to a wider audience, so ensure your entry is clear and unambiguous and conveys the information you want it to.

Box 9: Ten tips for good record keeping

1. Remember, your entry will be read by a wider audience, so it needs to:
   - be as brief as possible, but include all relevant details;
   - be clearly written;
   - state what you intended;
   - if the entry is lengthy, think about using headings to signpost the reader to important sections.
2. Write your entry so that someone reading it can understand what you mean and act upon any instructions for clinicians on the next shift/next day, etc.
3. Avoid 'sloppy' language that doesn't actually convey what has been happening, e.g. terms like 'unsettled' or 'threatening'. Explain what the person was doing and saying and exactly what you have observed.
4. Where clinical decisions have been made, e.g. changes in prescribed observations, explain the reasons for your decisions.
5. Describe the events that led to an incident. An extra sentence can be like 'gold dust' in helping the reader understand what happened and, importantly, why it happened.
6. Do not make personal comments in your entries that may be insulting or unnecessarily distressing to service users should they have access to their records. However, do not censor what needs to be written to be explicit about risk and other important issues because others will read what you have written. The important thing is to ensure it is written professionally and evidenced by being fact-based or by an impression drawn from a valid hypothesis (see below).
7. When you are expressing your impression/intuition to a risk you should clearly state this as opposed to fact-based evidence.
8. Record what you explained to the patient, i.e. their rights under the Mental Health Act. Also, if someone lacks capacity to make a safety care plan, make sure this is recorded.
9. Being explicit about key questions you have asked during a risk assessment can be useful in communicating how the information emerged during the interview.
10. Your RIO entries should be recorded within the span of your duty or, if in a crisis, at the earliest opportunity and no later than first thing the following day (O'Brien and Hart 2013).

References and selected bibliography

Appleby, L., Shaw, J., Kapur, N., Windfuhr, K., Ashton, A., Swinson, N. and While, D. (2006) *Avoidable Deaths: A Five Year Report of the National Confidential Inquiry Into Suicide And Homicide by People with Mental Illness*. Manchester: University of Manchester.

Bennewith, O., Gunnell, D., Peters, T.J., Hawton, K. and House, A. (2004) 'Variations in the hospital management of self-harm in adults in England: observational study', *British Medical Journal,* 328: 1108–09.

Breeze, J.A. and Repper, J. (1998) 'Struggling for control: the care experiences of "difficult" patients in mental health services', *Journal of Advanced Nursing*, 28: 1301–11.

Casement, P. (1985) *On Learning From the Patient*. London: Routledge.

Department of Health (2005) *Mental Capacity Act*. London: Department of Health.

Department of Health (2010) *See, Think, Act: Your Guide to Relational Security*. London: Department of Health.

Doyle, M. and Dolan, M. (2006) 'Predicting community violence from patients discharged from mental health services', *British Journal of Psychiatry*, 189: 520–26.

Gamble, C. and Curthoys, J. (2004) 'Psychosocial interventions', in Norman, I. and Ryrie, I. (eds) *The Art and Science of Mental Health Nursing: A Textbook of Principles and Practice*. Oxford: Oxford University Press.

Hamolia, C.D. (2005) 'Preventing and managing aggressive behaviour', in Stuart, G. and Laraira, M.T. (eds) *Principles and Practice of Psychiatric Nursing*. St Louis: Elsevier Mosby.

Hart, C. (2013a) *Working Effectively as a Primary Nurse*. London: South West London and St George's Mental Health NHS Trust.

Hart, C (2013b) *The SAFE Model of Nursing in a Psychiatric Intensive Care Unit*. London: South West London and St George's Mental Health NHS Trust.

Hillard, R. and Zitek, B. (2004) *Emergency Psychiatry*. New York: McGraw-Hill.

Maden, T. (2007) *Treating Violence: A Guide to Risk Management in Mental Health*. Oxford: Oxford University Press.

O'Brien, J. and Hart, C. (2013) *Clinical Risk Assessment and Risk Management*. London: South West London and St George's Mental Health NHS Trust.

Onyenaobiya, A. and Hart, C. (2013) 'Intensive personal support as an alternative to enhanced observations', Unpublished paper.

Ritter, S. (1989) *Bethlem Royal and Maudsley Hospital Manual of Clinical Psychiatric Nursing Principles and Procedures*. London: HarperCollins.

Van Heeringen, C. and Maruia, A. (2003) 'Understanding the suicidal brain', *The British Journal of Psychiatry,* 183: 282–84.

Wheeler, M. (2012) *Law, Ethics and Professional Issues for Nursing.* London: Routledge.

Williams, J.M.G, Crane, C., Barnhofer, T. and Duggan, D. (2005) 'Psychology and suicidal behaviour: elaborating the entrapment model', in Hawton, K. (ed.) *Prevention and Treatment of Suicidal Behaviour: From Science to Practice*. Oxford: Oxford University Press.

Note

1   For nurses involved in this process there is a secondary benefit, in that this kind of active work, not just in William's care but also in his treatment, gives nurses a clearer role and greater degree of authority to go with the responsibility they often have.

Summary and conclusions

This *Pocket Guide* has detailed the key issues about the practice of risk assessment and risk management in the area of mental health. Nonetheless, as was stated in the introduction, it has not set out to cover the entire evidence base or theory behind such practice and these are areas of knowledge that you should explore further. It is both a necessary and rewarding area of study, which requires continual application given the changing evidence base and advances in knowledge.

Gaining expertise in risk assessment and risk management, however, requires practice and although this needs to take place under close supervision initially, levels of expertise will only occur through the application of your experience and knowledge in clinical situations. In other words, there is no substitute for *doing*. Crucially, you should always remember the complexity and difficulty of this work, and whether you perceive yourself as being at the novice or expert end of the spectrum you won't always get it right, and can never know everything about the patient and the risks they face. Don't be afraid to ask for help, and remember clinical supervision is essential.

The statistics in Part 2 are there for your reference and highlight some important information and clinical risk factors. These cannot be used, however, as an alternative to a comprehensive assessment of the individual sitting in the room with you. The lists, tables and information boxes are not there to be 'ticked off' during an assessment but should act both as prompts and to provide a framework and structure for the assessment. They should stimulate your curiosity, willingness to carefully listen and think, helping you phrase your next question from an informed perspective but still based on what you have just heard the person say.

To quote an old and dear friend, always think about 'need to know and nice to know'. You have limited time, so make sure you have gained the essential information from the assessment to enable you to come up with the best possible risk management plan. If you're aware that you haven't got that yet, plan how you will make sufficient time and what contingency plan is required until you have.

Again, it must be emphasised that even the most robust assessment and management of risk cannot always prevent tragedies. Delving into all areas of risk, hoping for the best and planning for the worst will allow you to manage the most obvious risks. Careful consideration of those 'What if…?' questions will help you plan for the less obvious. Nonetheless, something may happen to change the situation in ways impossible to predict, even if that is only a change in the person's thinking, and lead to a serious incident or even the person's death. Reviewing such an event, you may at least be able to take comfort from seeing you had done the best job possible and that the risk was genuinely unforeseen. This is very different from someone repeating a past act or following the logical conclusions of past events or things s/he had been threatening, without an adequate plan in place to address it.

While you will always seek to collaborate with the person and work with their agenda as much as possible, don't be afraid to treat when necessary. Risk management, in all the details of its specific interventions, is a treatment. The risk management plan should not be driven by available resources but the needs of the person with you. That is an essential part of your duty of care. Once risk has been identified, a coherent, reasoned plan to assess it must be put in place.

Hopefully, the clinical examples will help you think about and find your own voice and use it. Each patient will teach you not only about her/himself but also about the assessment process itself. What cannot be captured on the page is the moments you listen, look, think and then act, always in the interest of that person and any others who may be at risk as a consequence of her/his actions.

Index

absconding 108, 112–113
Accident and Emergency
    Department (A&E
    Departments) 38, 47, 144–
    148, 160, 161
actuarial approach 48–49
aggression 2, 32, 35, 36, 153
alcohol use (see also, substance
    misuse) 26, 27, 28, 30, 34,
    35, 37, 97, 122, 127, 128,
    129, 160
anger 32, 36, 69, 161
anxiety 2, 28, 52, 67, 70, 75–76,
    97, 146, 155
Aristotle 50
arousal 52, 71, 137
    physiological 32, 36, 90
    psychological 86
arrested flight model 138
assertiveness 126
attempted suicide 9, 17, 22, 27,
    121–122, 130
auditory hallucinations 26, 116,
    136
autism 21, 37

bereavement 28, 129, 130
biographical history 95, 98
body language 55–56, 60, 65, 67,
    69, 70, 109, 133
body space 36
boundaries 67, 72, 152

carers 50, 56–58, 93,
    108–109
care plan 9, 41, 42, 63, 110,
    139–150, 162

interventions 115, 139–142,
    146–149, 151, 163, 176
    principles of 141
    structure 142, 147
    templates 141
care planning approach [cpa] 139
caseloads 14, 16
checklists 9, 157
clinical supervision 16, , 47, 156,
    165
closing down 82–84
codewords 53
coercion 2, 62
cognitions 32
collaboration, level of 13, 61, 62,
    63, 123, 128, 140, 152, 156
collaborative approach 2, 10,
    61–62, 63, 140, 149, 151
command hallucinations 31, 36,
    125
communication 15, 16, 55–56, 61,
    63, 87, 109, 155
    non verbal 67–68
compassion 155
concordance 62
concreteness 87
confidentiality 16, 56, 108
confronting 80, 154
congruence 55, 60, 69
consistency 109, 141, 151, 155
containment 52, 53, 67, 69,
    70–71, 113, 152–153, 155
contingency planning 14, 125,
    157, 165
coping strategies 9, 28, 39, 40,
    130, 139, 148
courtesy 64

crisis plans 158, 160–161
cultural diversity 6

dangerousness to others (see risk
    to others)
de-escalation skills 153
depression 2, 21, 28, 29, 31, 105
diagnosis 16, 26, 28, 37, 38, 49
digression 59, 84–85
dissociation 19
documentation 16, 32, 92, 95,
    149, 161
drug use (see also substance
    misuse) 5, 26, 28, 35, 53, 97,
    108, 128
dynamic risk factors 15, 38

early warning signs 12, 113, 116,
    128, 157, 159
education and training 15, 16, 47,
    139
empathy 61, 64, 69, 70, 78, 87,
    88, 155
entrapment 138

facial expression 36, 55, 56, 59,
    67, 69–70, 94, 109, 133
family 10, 22, 28, 30, 37, 50, 53,
    56–58, 75, 96, 102, 124, 128,
    158
family tree 128
forensic history 1, 97, 128
formulation 1, 6, 48, 50, 51, 91,
    105, 128, 129–130, 135,
    139
frequency of risk 12, 114, 128
funnelling in (see questions, types
    of)
future risk factors 13, 38–39, 49,
    119, 123

general practitioners 47, 60
genuineness 74, 86–88, 105
Golden Gate Bridge 127

HCR-20 49, 93
history of presenting complaint 94
home assessments 52–53
homicide 31–35
hopelessness 27, 28, 29, 38, 112,
    137, 138
hostility 32, 36, 153

immediacy 11, 55, 114
impulsivity 18, 26, 31, 36, 119,
    122, 126–127
incongruence 60
inquiries 16, 56, 57
insight 62, 106, 110, 111
instinct (see intuition)
intent 12, 17, 20, 27, 28, 36, 114,
    121, 137, 161
interpreter 6
interview structure 1, 17, 69, 72,
    93, 165
intuition 50, 60, 162

jargon 72
Johari's Window 110–111

labelling 31
loss 28, 30, 129, 138

medication 18, 23, 37, 75, 108,
    113, 141, 148, 151, 162
mental capacity 136–138, 162
Mental Capacity Act (2005) 136
Mental Health Act 1983 (as
    amended in 2007) 62, 129,
    138, 148, 162
mental health assessment 93–98

mental state examination
102–105, 128
mirroring 65, 70
motivation 17, 75, 94, 114, 123
negative attitudes 59–60
negotiation 64, 97, 105, 139, 142,
146, 148
NICE Guidelines on Self Harm 22
non compliance 16, 35, 37

observations 59
offenders 30, 33
pacing 64–65, 70

paramedics 47
parasuicide 17
patterns 11, 112
peer influence 126
personality disorder 16, 34, 37, 38,
129
phronesis 50, 60
positive risk taking 136, 147,
155–157
potential risk 11, 13–14, 19, 30,
38, 49, 52–54, 105, 108,
113–115, 120, 129, 136–137
PRN medication 151
prisoners (see offenders)
problem solving 81, 105, 126, 138
protective factors 30–31, 39, 122,
129, 130, 135, 140
Psychiatric Intensive Care Units
[PICU] 113, 138
psychosis 2, 28, 34–35, 37, 76, 84,
89, 101, 105, 111, 118, 119,
125, 126, 133, 138, 151
psychosocial assessment 22

questions, types of 72–75, 84,
115, 120, 123, 125, 126

closed 73–74
funnelling in 73–74
leading 89
multiple 89
open 73–74
opting out 98

rapid assessment 16, 127–128
rapport 9, 61, 63–65, 86, 102,
118, 120
re-assessment 36, 37, 115,
128–129, 149
recentness 10
record keeping (see
documentation)
recovery 141, 147, 148, 149, 156
referrals 39, 47, 51–52, 54–55,
129
reflection 78
relapse profile 5, 11, 158–170
relational management 16
resources 14, 16, 55, 105, 135,
166
respect 54, 87–88
rigidity 127
risk assessment tools 2, 39, 48, 93
risk factors 1, 10, 11, 20, 37–42,
48, 55, 124–126, 128,
130–131
external 107–109
individual 15
organisational 14, 139
team 15
and homicide 35
and violence 36–37
and suicide 27–30
risk, levels of 39–42
risk management plan 1, 13,
37–38, 40, 41, 46, 48, 50, 51,
52, 58, 63, 73, 92, 108–111,

118, 120, 123, 124, 125, 128,
131, 135, 138, 140–153, 156,
160, 162, 165–166
and families/carers 58, 108–109
risk, planning 12–13, 31, 119,
122, 126
risk profile 38, 126
risk, to others 2, 31, 36, 98–99,
113, 116–121, 138, 150–153

safety care plan (see risk
management plan)
scenario planning 111, 112–115,
124
schizophrenia 26, 34, 35
and homicide 34
seclusion 151–153
seeking clarification 75–77
self awareness 60
self disclosure 87, 88
self rating 50, 106–107
self-harm 1, 2, 17–22, 28, 30,
31–32, 37, 60, 113–114, 122,
125, 126, 148, 156
at risk groups 21
definition 9, 17
different age groups 20–21
gender and sexuality 6, 21
hospital admissions 20
impulsivity 127
intent 12, 121–122
locus of control 125
methods 18, 20
prognosis 22
rates 20
relationship to suicide 22,
27–30, 121
repeated 19, 20
risk assessment 11, 60, 121
risk management 148, 156

sexual abuse 21, 97
young people 21
semi structured interview 9
severity 11, 114, 138
sexual abuse 6, 21, 97
social skills 126
solution focused approach 81
stable risk factors 38
static risk factors 37–38
stress 18, 19, 26, 28, 38, 75,
113–114, 118, 125–126
structured clinical assessment (see
structured professional
judgement)
structured professional judgement
48
substance misuse 26, 34, 38, 39,
108, 111, 113, 119, 122,
135
suicidal thoughts 1, 2, 23, 27,
28, 91–92, 105, 125, 148,
150
suicide 1, 2, 17–23, 28–29, 108,
113, 121, 148
assessment of 31
and clinical risk indicators
27–29
definition 17
and formulation 130
and impulsivity 126–127
inquiries 16, 57
intent 121
locus of control 125
and men 23–26
and mental capacity 137
and mental illness 26
methods 27
planning 28, 31, 38
protective factors 30
rates 22–26, 30

and substance misuse 26
and women 22–23, 24–26
and young people 23
summarising 86

team organisation 14
telephone triage 50, 109
therapeutic relationship 63–64
therapeutic risk taking (see positive
    risk taking)
tick box (see checklists)
treatment plans 16
triage assessment 37, 47–48

unstructured clinical approach 48

violence 2, 31–32, 113, 114,
    118–119, 153
  and mental illness 34–35,
    98–102
  and risk assessment 53, 97,
    101–102, 111
  and risk factors 36-38

warning signs 12, 126, 128, 159
weapons, use of 36, 51, 53, 97,
    108, 119–120